ADVANCE PRAISE

"Kim is a perfect example of someone who makes a difference. *Fear Not, Angels Are Summed* is so compelling that I didn't put the book down until I finished the last page!"

—**Stephen DiMuzio**, Interior Designer,
Owner of Stephanie's of Stone Harbor

"Kim's story is an amazing journey through her life and her ability to use her faith to survive. I could not put the book down—so many emotional, funny, and inspiring moments!"

—**Carole Georges**, Retired VP, People's United Bank

"Providing hope for others, *Fear Not, Angels Are Summed* tackles an incredibly traumatic, life-altering accident with gripping details that make the book hard to put down. A story of resilience and recovery and a must-read for anyone in the midst of or recovering from trauma."

—**Heidi Ramsbottom**, Ph.D., Clinical Psychologist,
Center for Psychological Health & Wellness

"Kim's normal suburban life with her husband and three kids was turned upside down by a freak accident that could happen to any of us. Her trials and tribulations tested her tenacity, like God tested Job. Surviving the accident, 50 orthopedic surgeries, cancer, loss of job, moving and more were not enough to make her, or her family, give up. This personal story will inspire you to use your own will power, supported by those who care for you, to turn such negatives into a positive—to never lose hope and to turn it all around."

—**Dror Paley**, MD, FRCSC, Orthopedic Surgeon, Director, Paley Orthopedic and Spine Institute, West Palm Beach, Florida

"One word—BRAVO! I commend Kim Shipe for her bravery and sincerity in sharing her life's inspiring and incredible journey. I laughed with her and then wept with her when her pain was unimaginable. Kim is brutally honest in recreating the events that led her to finally find peace and resolve the pain she so long endured. A MUST READ!"

—**Val Patrician**, Wildlife and Folk Artist

"Despite incomprehensible odds, this mighty woman, mother, nurse, and runner overcomes all things with her faith and the guidance of many Angels. *Fear Not, Angels Are Summoned* will bring you such encouragement to face any storm thrown at you! I was on the edge of my seat through the entire book and shouting for joy with Kim and her family at the last chapter!"

—**Dottie Drake**, RN and Owner of Miracle's Fitness Club

"*Fear Not, Angels Are Summoned* recalls one woman's unbelievable journey that began as a typical day and ended by changing her and her family's lives forever. I found myself laughing at times, crying at others, and reflecting long after each chapter. Shipe's book is a mesmerizing, humble account of one woman's ability to see the Angels, even when she finds herself in life's darkest moments. A truly inspiring book."

—**Cyndie Veillette**, Special Education Instructor, Region 15 Schools, Massage Therapist, and Energy Worker

"I've worked as a counselor in the mental health and addiction field for over twenty years and have come to believe that faith and trust in God are the best predictors for healing, recovery, and good mental health. Kim's remarkable story describes how she transformed fear, pain, and suffering into faith, healing and an unshakeable belief and trust in God. She demonstrates how, by drawing on the love around us and from our Creator, we gain the stamina to maintain the tremendous effort and fortitude necessary for such a spiritual metamorphosis."

—**Patricia E. Meade**, MC, LPC, LISAC

"Kim Shipe's personal narrative captures the soul of a woman surviving numerous tragic events. The importance of love, family, friends, and faith provide the building blocks for her happiness!"

—**John Mudry**, Educational Consultant
and former School Principal

"A captivating testimony of tragedy and healing. Kim forges a sense of faith despite incredible odds."

—**Abby Hunsburger**, Retired Day Care Teacher for
the Child Development Center at the Reading Hospital

"I found *Fear Not, Angels Are Summed* to be thoroughly engaging. It had me laughing and in tears while thinking of my own life experiences. Kim frames this book with heart and soul. What an incredible human being!"

—**Jan Pouncey**, Retired Legal Assistant

"*Fear Not, Angels Are Summoned* is written through an act of love and witness to 'the Gospel.' In it one will find some of the unexpected ways God intervenes in the chaotic and most tragic moments of our lives. Kim Shipe's memoir articulates how the love of Christ surrounds us and brings us to healing and wholeness."

—**Rev. Nanette Christofferson**,
MDIV Fuller Theological Seminary, ELCA Pastor

"Kim's inspiring life story immediately draws you into the battle she faces between good and evil. She unknowingly invites evil in with her trusting, free spirit, and her desire to please others. She overcomes the darkness with the help of a newfound, unexpected friend who teaches her boundaries through example. She's a soul searching for purpose and truth. How a person can recover physically and spiritually from the horrific traumas in her life can only be done with Grace and help from above."

—**Karen Ord**, Rachel's Vineyard,
Retreat Coordinator, Phoenix, Arizona

FEAR NOT, ANGELS ARE SUMMONED

We all have a story to tell; & I hope that the story of my life inspires you. God bless you. Love, Kim

FEAR NOT, ANGELS ARE SUMMONED

Kem L Shipe

HOW ONE WOMAN OVERCAME UNIMAGINABLE SUFFERING TO LIVE A LIFE OF JOY

KIM L. SHIPE

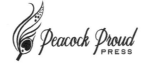

Peacock Proud
PRESS

Fear Not, Angels Are Summoned: How One Woman Overcame Unimaginable Suffering to Live a Life of Joy

Copyright © 2023 by Kim L. Shipe

First Published in the USA in 2023 by Peacock Proud Press, Phoenix, Arizona

ISBN 978-1-957232-09-6 Hardback
ISBN 978-1-957232-10-2 Paperback
ISBN 978-1-957232-00-3 eBook

Library of Congress Control Number: 2022921521

Editors
Laura L. Bush, PhD, peacockproud.com
Charles Grosel, write4success.net

Cover
Jena Gribble, blushcactus.com

Interior Layout
Medlar Publishing Solutions Pvt Ltd., India

Portrait Photographer
Greg DiGiovanni, photosbydigiovanni.com

I dedicate this book to The Lord, for completely healing me in His time and for sending the Angels to us. Thank you for Your healing mercies and for allowing me to continue to hear Your tender voice as You whisper in my ear. May I live out my life serving You!

I also dedicate this book to my husband, Rod Shipe, and our three children: Jason Shipe, Adam Shipe, and Sarah Pouncey. Without your unending support, encouragement, prayers, and dedication, I could have never done it! You guys are my heroes and just saying "Thank you" will never be enough!

TABLE OF CONTENTS

Preface . . . . *xv*

PART I – THE ACCIDENT

1 A Typical Day   3

2 Angels Are Summoned 15

PART II – ARMY BRAT

3 On the Move. 29

4 Dad Goes to Vietnam 41

5 Mustered Out 49

6 Innocence Lost 67

7 Saved by the New Kid in Town. 83

8 High School Girls Just Want to Have Fun 89

9 Falling for the Marlboro Man 101

10 Sweet Revenge 115

PART III – LIFE REBOOTED

11 Baseball with Barb 121

12 Good Things Come to Those Who Wait 125

13 This One's a Keeper 133

14 I Make a Career 137

15 Alcoholism, PTSD, and My Codependent Family 145

16 We Go to Rehab. 157

17 Our Family Grows: A Boy and a Girl 163

18 Life is Good 173

19 An Unsettling Time 183

PART IV – FALLOUT FROM THE ACCIDENT

20 A Night of Trauma Surgery. 191

21 Surgery, Pain, Puke, Repeat 195

22 More Messengers 201

23 The Community Cares 207

24 Disappointment Prevails 217

25 A Brief Homecoming 223

26 Respite Cut Short. 229

27 Surgery and Fireworks 241

28 Physical Rehabilitation 247

29 Going Home for Good. 253

30 Challenges and More Challenges. 261

31 I've Never Seen *This* Before. 271

32 Lose the Limp. 275

33 The End is in Sight ... Or Is It? 277

34 Surgery Resumed 287

35 False Heart Attack 291

PART V – THE ROAD TO HEALING
FAITH, FORGIVENESS, FUN (AND LOTS OF THERAPY)

36 Happiness Is a Choice. 307

37 Faith: Let Go and Let God 315

38 Forgiveness: The Gift You Give Yourself. 321

39 I Try My Hand at Business 333

40 The Joy of Running Again. 337

41 If You Can't Take Wing, Try a Parachute. 341

Afterword. 347

Notes 351

Acknowledgments. 353

About the Author 357

PREFACE

This will not be an easy book to read. I know that because it was not an easy book to write. I've experienced a great deal more trauma than most people—rape, a horrendous accident in which I almost lost my legs, a bilateral mastectomy for breast cancer. These were difficult to go through when they happened, they were difficult to re-experience as I wrote about them, and no doubt they will be difficult to read about. For that I apologize. But I don't want your pity. I'm not a victim. Victims haven't healed. I've healed.

I have not written this book to raise myself up because of what I've suffered. What happened to me happened to me—it could have happened to anyone. I'm nobody special. Better yet, I *am* somebody special, just as we are all somebody special in the eyes of God. So really, I've written this book to remind myself of that, of how far I've come, of how God and his Angels have been with me every step of the way. And I've written it to let you know that even in the midst of unspeakable pain, there is joy to be found. If my story can help even one person get through a rough patch, then it was worth the time and angst it took to write (and the time it takes to read, I hope). Thank you for bearing with me.

PART I

THE ACCIDENT

Be strong and courageous.
Do not be afraid.
Do not be discouraged.
For the Lord your God
will be with you wherever you go.

—Joshua 1:9

CHAPTER 1

·····························

A TYPICAL DAY

It was May 1, 2002, a typical morning for the Shipe family. My husband, Rod, was out of town. I didn't expect him back until later that evening. Once out of bed, I lowered the silhouette blinds and looked in awe as the morning sun peeked through the trees across the street. I grabbed my camera from the closet and snapped a few pictures in a vain attempt to capture God's splendor. Then I woke the kids. They hurried to my bedroom and together we watched the sunrise, which they agreed was worth getting out of bed for. I was pleased I could share the beauty of the morning with my children before the chaos of the day took over. Before they left, I remembered that it was May first.

"Do you know what today is?" I asked the two kids.

"Wednesday," Adam said, the literal fifteen-year-old.

"Yes, but it's also May 1, May Day. Do you know what May Day meant when I was your age?"

"No, what did May Day mean when you were our age?" Sarah rolled her eyes. She was twelve. Not another Mom story!

I told them how May Day was a celebration of spring, of rebirth, one of those elementary school traditions no one honored any more. How we nominated a May Queen, someone who was not only pretty but also nice to others. How we didn't have classes that day. How a carnival was set up on the playground with games to play. How we could win prizes or tickets. How we exchanged the tickets for goodies to eat: cotton candy, snow cones, penny candy, and other carnival foods. How the celebration lasted all day.

The main attraction was the May Dance, I explained further, for which we practiced for weeks. Each child held a colorful ribbon attached to the top of the Maypole. Once the music started, we walked clockwise around the pole as we lifted our ribbon above the first child's ribbon and then below the next child's ribbon and so on. We continued around the Maypole until we ran out of ribbon. By the end of the dance, we had weaved a colorful pattern and learned to appreciate teamwork. It was a proud moment for us when our parents joyfully clapped at the result. I always spotted Mom in the crowd, but Dad was usually on military deployment.

Although I'm sure Adam wanted to rush out of the room to get into the shower first, he stopped and listened respectfully. Sarah, on the other hand, inched her way towards the double doors. She was more interested in picking out the perfect outfit for school.

I lingered briefly in the fond childhood memories, and then released them to the morning's business. "Get your showers. I'll see you downstairs."

I paused at the window to take in the scene one more time. It felt serene, almost surreal, too beautiful and perfect not to pause and appreciate it one last time. A glance at the alarm clock, though, told me I needed to hurry.

After a quick shower, I dressed and rushed downstairs to get breakfast going.

It was all so typical, so routine.

My kids and my husband were my entire life. I was a caregiver, just as my own mom had been when I was growing up. She not only took great care of us, but she was a Florence Nightingale to everyone she met. She genuinely cared for others and had a heart of gold.

We hurried through a breakfast of milk and cereal. I took out our Weimaraner, Madison, one last time while the kids packed their bookbags and headed to my black Volvo sedan. Even after I backed out of the garage, I took note of the crystal blue sky that stretched on forever. Not a single cloud hung in the sky that morning, and it reminded me that spring had finally arrived in New England. I opened my car window to feel the gentle warm breeze and take in the scent of the blooming flowers. *Just wonderful*, I thought. *Magnificent.*

I pulled out of our development in Southbury, Connecticut, and down Georges Hill Road. Adam's school bus picked him up a short distance ahead at the commuter lot. At fifteen, he still attended a private school in Waterbury. The bus was on time. As he was ready to climb the steps, he turned and gave us the family "I love you" sign. When the kids were younger, our "I love you" sign was to point to our eye, then our heart, and then to the other person. As the kids got older, they worried other kids might laugh, so they changed it to a simple hook motion with our index fingers. We never left each other without exchanging the sign.

Sarah switched to the front seat, and we headed towards her middle school. She had also attended the private school in Waterbury, but after a year, she had begged us to let her to return to the public school, and we had agreed.

As we drove, Sarah remembered that she had a dental appointment that day at three. She had her first cavity and was afraid to get a filling. I assured her that it was no big deal, that many kids had cavities filled, but she wasn't buying it.

I reminded her that I would leave *my* school early to take her to the dentist. I was a nurse at the elementary school down the road. Since the middle school's day ended before the elementary school's, Sarah would take a bus to the elementary school. Then I would take her to her appointment. When we arrived at her school, I told her again it would be all right, and finally she left the car, turned, and hooked her finger for "I love you." I returned the sign and smiled before I pulled away.

Our three kids had always seemed to be part of our marriage. When Rod and I married in 1979, I was blessed with a seven-year-old stepson, Jason. Then almost seven years later we had our second son, Adam, and two-and-a-half years after that we were blessed with a daughter, Sarah. I always wanted children. Two boys and a girl seemed perfect.

I loved being a mom, but it wasn't always easy. Parenthood doesn't come with an instruction booklet. Rod and I tried our best, in a loving manner, and I think we did pretty well. Over the years we involved the kids in preschool, dance lessons, gymnastics, play dates, soccer, T-ball, softball, baseball, basketball, art lessons, summer camps, surfing, golf, and tennis. Rod coached the kids' basketball teams, and I was the scorekeeper. For less structured activities, we had bridle paths nearby that Rod and I liked to run on with Madison, while the kids rode their bikes. We always tried to listen to the kids when they spoke and let them know their feelings were important to us.

Despite the hectic morning, I made it to work on time. The elementary school was also in Southbury, a classic rural, middle-class New England town with loads of charm. In most households, both parents worked, and some commuted as far as New York City on the trains that passed through nearby Danbury.

It was not going to be a typical day at school. I had another nurse covering the office and my 500 students because I was helping the staff register next year's kindergarten class. My job was to screen the future kindergarteners and collect their immunization and health records from their parents. Despite work commitments, the parental involvement at the school was exceptional. I had an excellent rapport with parents and a special connection with the children. I loved the job's regular schedule and felt blessed to have it. It was the polar opposite of one of my previous jobs as a critical care nurse, which often required me to work weekends and nights and had been a nonstop adrenaline rush. I was in my third year, and I intended to stay there until retirement.

The screenings were back-to-back-to-back, and the morning flew by without any issues. At lunch I couldn't stop thinking about Sarah and how nervous she had been about her dentist appointment. She was intensely afraid of medical procedures. I always tried to reassure my children by explaining the procedures as factually and frankly as possible to lessen their fear, but nothing in my arsenal was working with Sarah. Before I returned to the afternoon screenings, I said a quick prayer for her.

The afternoon screenings were also uneventful. I finished well in advance of two-thirty, when Sarah's bus dropped her off. We drove less than a mile down Main Street to the dentist's office. I talked the entire drive to distract her, but I still had to coax her into the office while I held her sweaty hand. I walked her to the dental chair, explained her fears to the dentist and his hygienist, and remained with her until they were ready to start. I told her that I had to pick up Adam at the bus stop, and then the two of us would return to pick her up. I gave her a quick, "I love you" sign before I left.

Adam and I returned just as the dentist finished up. I was so relieved to see Sarah smiling. She told me it wasn't as horrible as she had imagined. I told her I was proud of her. "Let's celebrate!" I called out. "Who wants ice cream?"

"We do!" the kids responded.

We headed towards the car. "Where are we going, Mom?" Sarah asked.

"Denmo's."

"Can we get food, too?" Adam asked, the perpetually hungry teenager.

"Sure," I said as I unlocked the car. We didn't expect Rod home until after dinner, so we didn't need to rush. Sarah got into the back seat after Adam held the front seat forward, then Adam sat in the passenger seat. Even though we had only a two-minute drive down Main Street to the outdoor take-out restaurant, as soon as I started the car, Adam began channel surfing on the radio.

From the back seat Sarah complained: "I hate that station and hate that song and since I'm crammed in the back seat, I should be able to pick the music!"

"No, the person in the front seat picks the music," Adam retorted.

"I just had a dentist appointment. I should be in charge."

"What're you going to do about it?" he said in the taunting teenage voice he saved for his sister. "I'm in control." He pressed the buttons one after the other to prove it.

"STOP!" I yelled. "ENOUGH IS ENOUGH. I'm so tired of you two fighting. Today the driver picks the music and I pick nothing." I reached over and turned off the radio as I pulled into Denmo's parking lot, a front row space, just to the right of the ordering windows.

Usually, the kids placed and paid for their own orders, but that day, I wasn't happy with them. "I am so disgusted with how often you fight. Both of you just stay in the car." I turned toward Adam. "What do you want, Adam?"

"One hot dog with chili and cheese and fries smothered with chili and cheese," he said.

"Sarah, what about you?"

"One plain hot dog and fries with cheese on the side."

I repeated their orders twice to make sure I got them. "Okay, I want you to watch for the food, because I'm going to need help carrying it. That's the only time you can get out of the car." I slammed the door behind me.

I picked the line closest to the car because it was the shortest. *I guess I'll get a small dish of vanilla ice cream for me. Nah, maybe a medium. I'm sort of hungry.* Then I repeated the kids' orders in my head so I wouldn't forget.

I lost my train of thought when I heard a woman yell at her children somewhere behind me. *A lot of that going on today,* I thought. *Okay,* I continued. *Two orders of fries, one with cheese on the side and the other smothered with chili and cheese. Two hot dogs, one plain and the other with chili and cheese and a medium cup of vanilla ice cream.*

I got it. My line was moving slowly, but I didn't care. I was next. The other cashier called out something I didn't understand. When I looked her way, she waved me over. Her line was empty.

I switched lines and recited my order. The cashier tapped it into the register, then read it back to me. I told her it was correct. She gave me the total. I reached into my purse for my wallet, paid her in cash. After she handed me the change, I placed it in my wallet, and closed my purse.

Before I could step away from the window, two things happened virtually simultaneously. It was only later that I could untie the knot.

I heard what sounded like a gunshot at close range, and then I was hit from behind by a wave-like force that propelled me forward. I hit something hard, and for a moment I was suspended in time, thinking nothing really. Then the wave broke, and I heard people screaming. The mom was still yelling at her children, now much louder, and with the kind of terror I recognized as that of a mother fearing her children were in danger. "Get in the car now," she yelled.

It occurred to me that someone must have been shot. *Who was shot?* I wondered. *Someone should help them.* Then I remembered that something had hit me hard. *Is it me? Did I get shot? OH, MY DEAR GOD, NO, IF I WAS SHOT, DON'T LET ME DIE IN FRONT OF MY KIDS. Please, God, no,* I silently prayed, and as I did so, I was moving again, this time very slowly and backwards. Against all odds, I found myself sitting on the hood of a car. The voice in my head was trying to make sense of what was going on. *I'm not shot. I've been hit by a car and pushed through the front of the restaurant, and I just rolled out of the building. Am I all right?* I looked down at my legs to take inventory. I was wearing pants, but within the pantlegs my right foot seemed to be backwards, and the front of my left foot was twisted sideways facing my right foot. Both legs were swinging side to side and spinning in semi-circles. *My legs are going to fall off! Oh my God help me!*

I looked up and this time *I* was screaming. "Oh my God, my legs! Call 911. Someone call 911!"

From inside the building a girl shouted, "We just called 911!"

I looked around. Everyone inside the building was staring at me. No one was working, they were just standing still, stupefied by what they had witnessed. I looked at my legs again, and screamed, "My legs. Oh my God, my legs! My legs." Fearing greater injury, I thought that maybe I should get off the hood of the car. This didn't make sense, but I was convinced that I had to get off the hood of that car. Slowly, I scooted to the right, my legs swinging and twisting even more. I slowed down, afraid my legs would fall off if I moved too fast. When I finally reached the edge of the hood, I pushed off with my arms and jumped. I wasn't making any sense. At the same time I feared that my legs were falling off, I thought they'd be able to hold me up after a jump like that. I just had to get off that car. While I was in midair, a man reached out and caught me, then held me up, my legs flailing. I looked into his eyes and screamed, "Oh my God, my legs are going to fall off!"

In my ear he whispered, "Your children are here, and they're very upset. Please try to calm down, for their sake. They can hear everything. Please calm down."

My eyes met his and I knew he was right. I didn't want to die in front of my children, nor did I want their last memory of me to be my screaming in fear and pain. "Okay," I said. "Okay."

Later I learned that my savior was Carl Cruis, a patron at the restaurant that day. He had been waiting for his hot dog, and when he saw me scooting along the hood, he dashed around the back of the car to catch me when I pushed off.

As a critical care nurse, I was trained to respond to an emergency on a moment's notice. I did that now, except I was the victim and it was my emergency. It was as if I physically left my body to direct my own care from afar. This was the big fight, the fight for my life. I had to do whatever I needed to do to stay alive. I don't think the first responders had seen anything like it before.

The Southbury Ambulance Association had recently relocated next door to Denmo's. An EMT named Monique was the only one on site just then. Everyone else was responding to an accident at the other end of Main Street. She joined us beside the car, where Carl held me. She assessed the situation, then gave detailed instructions to Carl on how she would take hold of one side of my body and Carl would hold the other side until they could get a blanket to lay me down on. That's when the first police officer, Don, arrived on the scene. He took Carl's place and held me up on my right side. For my part, I was alert, cooperative, and calm, and I helped make decisions. I had cried out for God so many times that I felt He answered me. He was right there with me giving me exactly what I needed.

One of the stranger things about that very strange day was that at this point I wasn't feeling pain. It takes a body time to process such a catastrophic injury. Adrenaline pumped through my body and my heart raced from the excitement. In the back of my mind, though, I knew that once the pain hit, it would be horrific, unlike anything I had ever experienced and that no amount of medication would relieve it completely. I tried not to think about that.

Meanwhile, I figured I should get some practical things taken care of. "It's obvious I'm going to have surgery tonight," I said to Officer Don. "I'm going to take my jewelry off. Can you put it in the zippered part of my purse?"

"Sure," Officer Don said.

I took off my earrings, then my necklace, and finally my rings. Officer Don helped me put everything in my purse, then he zippered the small section closed. As I looked in my purse, I remembered that I had cashed a check for $36.00 that belonged to my daughter's AAU basketball team, which my husband coached. I pulled out the sealed bank envelope and showed it to him. "This cash belongs to the AAU basketball team my daughter plays on, and my husband is their coach. $36.00. Could you please make sure my husband knows it's in my purse?"

"Yes, Ma'am," he said.

My kids! Where are my kids? I looked around, but I couldn't see them. Many people now surrounded us. There were more police officers as well as another EMT, but no ambulance yet.

Someone brought over a blanket, opened it, and spread it on the ground.

Ever so gently, Monique and Officer Don lowered me onto the blanket. Monique assured me the ambulance and additional help were on the way.

Her hands free, Monique got to work. "Your legs are twisted and turned in the wrong direction. I'm concerned that the circulation to your feet is restricted. If you'll bear with me, one by one I'm going to turn your legs in the right direction, okay?"

"Yes," I said. I gripped Don's hand and took a deep breath. "I'm ready." I expected excruciating pain to begin right about then, and I braced myself.

Slowly and carefully, she lifted and turned the first leg and positioned it horizontally on the blanket. Much to my amazement, I had no pain!

She looked into my eyes again and said, "Are you ready?" I nodded and took another deep breath. She supported the other leg and slowly lifted and turned it until it was untwisted, then she lowered it carefully onto the blanket. There was no pain this time either! Once I was settled, Officer Don asked me some basic questions, such as my name and address, and both he and Monique jotted down my responses. Even more police arrived, and several of them encircled the area where I was lying in yellow crime scene tape.

Another paramedic joined us, took one look at me, then turned to Monique and said, "I can't help. Sorry!"

"Why not?"

"I can't look at those legs again!" he said, and ran off with his hand covering his mouth.

"Then find someone else!"

"*What?*" I thought. *He's a first responder. What if I didn't have pants on?*

As Monique took my blood pressure, I listened to two police officers a few feet away. The first one said, "Give the kids the car keys and tell them to drive home."

Did I just hear that correctly? Do they mean Adam and Sarah? From my position on the ground, I hollered, "Did I just hear you say you're going to give my kids the car keys and tell them to drive home?"

The police officer closest to me said, "Yes." He was surprised by my question. He must have thought I was out of it.

"Neither of them has a driver's license. And even if they did, do you really think they'd be able to drive home after this?" I pointed to the police officer and said, "You, find my kids and take them behind this building and tell them they have to stay there until you tell them they can leave."

Then I pointed to the officer he was talking to and said, "And you. You go back to them every five minutes and tell them I'm okay. Even if I die here, you tell them I'm okay. You got that?"

The officer looked at me as he said, "Yes, Ma'am."

I realized I hadn't seen the kids at all, although I knew they had seen me. I was grateful they were elsewhere at that moment. They must have seen the entire accident, since the last thing I told them was to watch me in case I needed help with the food. I wished I hadn't said that.

That was about the time I heard a siren approaching. Finally.

Once the ambulance arrived, a full crew got to work assisting Monique. Someone stuck an IV in my arm. Someone took my vitals. Several of them lifted me very carefully onto a litter, covered me with blankets, and loaded me into the ambulance.

Once I was inside, Officer Don peeked his head through the side door and said, "I'm so sorry this happened to you and your family. Is there anything else I can do?"

I looked into his concerned eyes. I knew my accident would affect all the responders for some time, and I wanted to ease the tension. "Yes, there is one thing. I never got my food. Can you get me a go bag?" I will never forget how the look in his eyes flashed from concern to panic, as if to say, *Are you serious?* I left him hanging only a few seconds before I laughed. I reached for his hand and said, "I'm kidding. Thanks for everything. Take care of my kids."

An EMT slammed the side door shut. The back doors had already been closed. Red lights flashed and sirens echoed down Main Street on our way to Waterbury Hospital.

······························

CHAPTER 2

ANGELS ARE SUMMONED

As soon as the ambulance left, the police told Adam and Sarah they could leave the back of the building where they had been instructed to wait. (I learned most of the details about the events I wasn't present for later from the different participants.) Sarah noticed a teacher she knew in the crowd. She walked over to her and said, "That was my mom who was just hit by a car."

"Oh, Sarah, I'm so sorry. What can I do for you and your brother?" The teacher's name was Diane.

"Um, could you take us to our friends' houses? Our dad is out of town."

"I'd be happy to."

Just then a sergeant from the Southbury Police Department approached them. Diane explained that she knew both children and didn't mind taking them to their friends' houses, since their dad was out of town. The officer asked each child where they planned to go, as well as for a phone number so he could make sure a parent was home there. He went to his patrol car to make the calls, then returned to let

Diane know that he had reached a parent at both homes and she was free to leave with the children.

Once in the car—Adam in the back seat, Sarah up front—the children spoke only to give directions. Adam was first. His friend, Ryan, lived in Woodbury, which was a few miles from Southbury. Ryan's father was the headmaster at Adam's school. When they arrived at Ryan's house, Adam turned to Diane and politely said, "Thank you for driving me to my friend's house."

"You're welcome, Adam, and I'm so sorry about your mom's accident."

"Thanks," was all he could say. Then he said, "Bye Sarah."

Sarah looked at Adam sadly and said, "Bye Adam."

Ryan had been waiting for Adam since they had received the call from the police officer. Once Adam was inside, Ryan's mom, who was also a registered nurse, asked him what had happened. He was still in shock and couldn't really talk about the accident. Instead, he got a piece of paper out of his backpack and drew a picture. Adam was quite the artist so I'm certain his drawing showed just how serious the accident had been. As a nurse, Ryan's mother understood how traumatized Adam must have been. I'll be forever grateful that she came through for Adam and our family on that awful day.

Next, Sarah instructed Diane on how to get to her best friend Lindsay's house. The girls played basketball together. Sarah kept quiet in the car. The accident was all she could think about. When Diane pulled into Lindsay's driveway, Sarah also said, "Thank you."

"You're welcome, Sarah."

Lindsay and her mom, Carole, came outside to meet Sarah. Diane knew Carole and Lindsay, so she got out of the car as well.

"What happened?" Carole asked Diane while Lindsay and Sarah started to talk.

By this time both girls had joined them, so Diane was careful about what she said. "Kim was hit by a car while standing at Denmo's."

"Oh no, what kind of injuries does she have?"

"Nothing life threatening. Possibly two broken legs," Diane said loud enough for the two young girls to hear. When the girls turned away, she met Carole's eyes and shook her head to indicate it was much worse than that.

Carole nodded, feeling queasy. Then she said, "Thanks for bringing Sarah to our house. The girls have a class trip tomorrow, so Sarah had planned to sleep over anyway."

"If there's anything else I can do ...." Then Diane got back into her car and backed out of the driveway.

Carole, Lindsay, and Sarah went into the house. Carole talked with Sarah a bit to calm her down, then thought she should call Rod to let him know what was going on.

Rod should have been somewhere between Pennsylvania and Connecticut by then, but in 2002, roaming cell phone reception wasn't very good. Sarah dialed his number, then handed the phone to Carole, but there wasn't an answer. For the next forty-five minutes, they repeated the same ritual until finally Rod answered his cell phone.

"Hi Dad, it's Sarah. I'm at Lindsay's house. Hold on for a minute. Her mom wants to talk to you."

Sarah handed the phone to Carole as if to say, I don't want to tell my dad.

"Hi Rod."

"Hi Carole, what's up?"

She took a deep breath and said, "Where are you?"

"Just passing the Danbury Mall on eighty-four."

"I have some bad news. Kim was in an accident at Denmo's today and was taken to the Waterbury Hospital. Both kids are okay, though. They weren't involved."

"Is Kim okay?" he asked.

"She might have broken at least one of her legs," she said. "But that's all I know."

"Is Adam at your house too?"

"No. Sarah said he went to Ryan's house."

"I'll call you later from the hospital once I get to see her. Is Sarah okay?"

"She was very upset when she got here, but we've talked with her, and now she seems a little better. Don't forget that tomorrow is their class trip to Boston. Let me know when we talk later if she should go on the trip or stay with you, okay?"

"Yes, I'll do that. Thanks Carole. Call me anytime Sarah needs me."

Rod was only about fifteen minutes from home. He stopped at the house to feed the dog and let her out, changed clothes, then headed to the hospital. He figured I'd be in the ER for a while before the specialists arrived.

Meanwhile Carole asked Sarah, "Where's your mom's car?"

"Still at Denmo's," she said.

"Do you have her keys?"

"In my backpack."

"Get them for me. Steve and I will get your mom's car and take it to your house."

When Steve and Carole got to Denmo's, they were shocked to see the damage as they pulled into the parking lot. Crime scene tape encircled the front of the building, which was caved in by the car whose back end stuck out from the hole it had made. The police were still working diligently at the scene, taking notes and measurements.

Carole drove my Volvo to our house. As she headed up Georges Hill Road, she saw Rod heading in the opposite direction to the hospital, his four-way hazard lights flashing urgently.

While all that was happening without my awareness, I faced some challenges of my own. Namely, that the pain my body had been holding off suddenly hit me as if I had run into a brick wall. It was instantly horrific. I moaned loudly and reached for my legs. It felt like someone was stabbing both legs over and over and over again while someone else was trying to rip my legs from the rest of my body. Before that day, I thought labor was going to be the worst pain I would ever experience. This pain made labor feel like a hangnail. And I knew it was only going to get worse!

The EMT, a woman, saw my face contort and asked, "Has the pain hit?"

"Yes," I whispered. "Really bad. Please give me something." I moaned loudly.

"I'll contact the ER doctor," she said. She got in touch with the team awaiting my arrival, and got an order for intravenous morphine, which she administered directly into my IV. I felt woozy, and the pain seemed to get more intense rather than less. I tapped on the side of the litter as I continued to moan. It was difficult to focus on anything but the intensifying pain. "Can't you give me more? That didn't touch it at all. Please, please give me anything."

"If your vitals are good, I can give you more. We'll be at the hospital in two minutes." She took my blood pressure, then my pulse, and she must have been satisfied, because then she pushed the rest of the medicine into the IV line. "We're at the hospital," she announced.

The pain was starting to ease a bit when the back doors of the ambulance flew open. The attendants lifted me out and rolled my gurney with urgency into a large trauma room where a team of nurses and a doctor had been waiting. Bright lights illuminated the space, which was circled by medical equipment and IV machines.

"Hello, Mrs. Shipe, we've been waiting for you. I'm Dr. Moss. We are going to work as a team to determine the extent of your injuries." Then to his team he said, "On three lift her onto the bed. One, Two, Three."

I screamed, loudly. I was experiencing such incredible pain and anything they tried to do involving my legs ratcheted that pain even higher than I could have imagined. "Please, please you have to give me something for the pain. The pain is incredible."

The doctor immediately gave an order for more morphine and one of the nurses retrieved it from their medicine cart and pushed it into my IV. My vision flickered so I closed my eyes. Another nurse put a second IV line in my arm as I lay motionless, trying to focus on slowing my breathing as the morphine worked its magic and the pain became less intense.

"Bear with us as we cut off your clothes," one of the nurses said.

First my shirt was cut and a gown was placed and snapped closed over my shoulders. My shoes were removed before my socks were cut off. Then they worked side-by-side to cut my pants off starting at the bottom of each leg. Suddenly the pain shot through the morphine and was so intense I screamed and begged them to stop. I even tried to grab their hands. When they worked anywhere near my legs, the pain was so bad it felt as if they were ripping my legs off, as if they were tearing my flesh and bones and blood vessels without mercy. "Please give me some pain meds that actually work, or give me anesthesia and send me to surgery, so I don't have to feel any more pain," I yelled at them. I screamed louder than I had ever screamed before. Until then I would NEVER have been anything but a quiet and cooperative patient, as any doctor or nurse would have wanted, but that day the pain was so intense I didn't give a damn how loud or rude or hysterical I sounded. I wanted them to know what they were doing to me, and I wanted them to stop.

"We'll cut as fast as we can, but we have to get your pants off before we can do anything else," said another of the nurses.

Before I could object, the cutting resumed. I yelled even louder as they approached the midcalf region. My exhausted body, shot through with adrenalin and morphine, trembled uncontrollably from head to toe as beyond all belief the intense pain got even more intense. My screams were now blood curdling. I simply didn't care who heard me, or what I screamed! I just desperately needed it to end, one way or another!

"Are you cold?" I heard someone ask.

With eyes closed and tears streaming down my face, I said, "No."

"Give her more morphine," the doctor said.

Another dose was pushed through as they made their last cuts on my pants.

"We're sending you for a CT scan and X-rays. One of our nurses will go with you." This was also the doctor.

Oh no, I thought, *my pain was finally easing and now more people are going to torture me! Fuck, just let me die*, I wanted to scream but I held back.

They moved me to the imaging room for a CT scan of my legs. Moving me onto and off the scanning table caused so much pain that I screamed each time. They also took x-rays of my legs and the intensity of pain was so severe when they arranged my body that all I could do was scream and shake violently from head to toe. The pain was growing even more intense. When we returned to the trauma room, the doctor gave orders for a higher dose of morphine.

The doctor moved closer to my face and said, "Mrs. Shipe, we're going to prep you for transfer to Yale New Haven Hospital. You need emergency orthopedic trauma surgery, and we can't do that here. I've already spoken to the trauma team at Yale, and they're prepping for you. You'll go directly into surgery. Do you have any questions?"

"Please write on the front of my chart that I am refusing all blood products."

"For religious reasons?" he asked.

"No, personal preference. But put it on my chart anyway!"

He didn't say anything else, so I assumed he did what I said.

"We need to put dressings around your legs. I know this will be painful. Please bear with us. If your vital signs are stable, we will continue to give you pain medication. We're getting everything ready now."

Oh, My Dear Lord God come to me now and give me your peace, was all I could think to pray before the torture began again.

The nurses worked as a team to get everything done as quickly as possible. Several nurses lifted my right leg without warning. I screamed in agony. *Why couldn't I just have died?* I said to myself. *It would have been so much easier.* I watched the faces of the nurses as they worked.

As a critical care nurse, I had stood in their shoes many times and felt the same way—the disbelief, the graphic reality, the pain and suffering. Could their efforts help? For how long? Would she live? Would she die? Would the suffering break her spirit? Another shot of pain stopped that line of thinking, my body shaking, contorting, as if it could twist away from the pain.

I screamed, "Pain medicine!" but they just kept working as I screamed. My arms flailed weakly as I grabbed at their hands again and again to get them to stop.

✦ ✦ ✦

Rod pulled into the ER parking lot, found a spot near the entrance. He walked rapidly, eager to get to me and hoping my legs weren't too bad. When the automatic doors flung open, he heard a bloodcurdling scream that was chillingly familiar. The nausea of panic hit Rod. He ran toward the screams. Before he could get into the trauma room, the emergency staff cut him off.

"Where are you going?" the guard asked.

"That's my wife screaming, and I want to see her now!"

"You can't go in there yet!"

"Why not?"

"The doctor needs to talk to you."

The screaming continued. "You can't stop me!"

"Please, wait here with the nurse and I'll get him for you."

Rod nodded and began pacing in horror and disbelief.

Within seconds, the doctor came out of the room, and spoke with kindness and empathy. He explained the severity of my injuries and that I had lost a great deal of blood. He told Rod I would need a trauma team that handled these types of injuries and they couldn't do that at this small community hospital. He explained he had already contacted Yale New Haven and their trauma team was prepared to take me directly into surgery.

"Okay. Got it. Can I please see her now?"

"Yes."

Rod ran into the room, and with tears in his eyes he leaned over and kissed my forehead. Then he took my hand and squeezed it and said, "It's going to be okay. They're taking you to Yale, and you'll have surgery tonight."

"I know. I know. But before they do, I want you to make a call for me. Adam has a friend, also Adam. His dad is an orthopedic surgeon. Please call him and make sure that whatever they plan for surgery is medically necessary. Okay? I need my legs, Rod." I closed my eyes against the pain of the effort to get that out.

"Yes, of course. Don't worry, Kim. I'll take care of it."

"Are the kids okay?"

"Yes. They're good. Adam is at Ryan's house. Sarah is at Lindsay's."

"I'm in so much pain," I confessed. "I don't know what to do!"

"Please give her more pain meds," Rod begged one of the nurses. "Don't make her suffer any more!"

An automatic blood pressure reading had just been taken. Since it was extremely high, more medicine was given.

I had a few more things to take care of with Rod. "All my jewelry is in my purse. I also cashed the check for the basketball team, and it's in a bank envelope in there too."

"Kim, it's okay. Stop worrying. It's not that important right now."

Someone entered the room and announced the ambulance had arrived.

Rod told the doctor, "I'm going to leave now so I can get to Yale ahead of the ambulance." Then Rod kissed me goodbye. "I'll see you in a few minutes, honey. I love you."

"I love you, too," I whispered in exhaustion.

The ambulance crew had already entered the room. One of the nurses gave a report to one of the EMTs. The EMTs lifted me onto their litter, covered me with a sheet and blanket as I moaned in pain. As the crew rolled me out of the trauma room, I hollered to the ER crew, "Goodbye and thanks for all you've done!"

I heard a faint, "Good luck," behind me.

The automatic doors opened to reveal the darkness of a night sky. All those hours lost to that black hole of pain. Once inside the ambulance bay, I was joined by the same female EMT who had brought me there. I had forgotten her name, but I figured at this point did it even matter?

"On a scale of one to ten how bad is the pain right now?" she asked.

"Twenty," I said.

"Okay," she said. "I'll get some vitals and see what the doctors at Yale want to give you."

The siren was so loud as we sped out of town and onto the highway, I didn't know how she could hear the instructions on the radio, but she must have been able to, because the next thing I knew she was injecting pain meds into my IV line. These meds didn't end the pain, but they did take some of the intensity away. Time had no meaning. Suddenly, without reason the intensity of pain shot up tenfold. I was shaking uncontrollably. My breathing was rapid and shallow, as if I was having a panic attack. I opened my eyes and begged for more medication.

She shook her head. "I can't give you anything. Your blood pressure is dropping. I'm only getting a palpable blood pressure of 80. I have to call the ER STAT." She got the ER doctor on her radio. "She is in extreme pain and requesting pain medicine, but I'm only getting a palpable BP of eighty. What should I do?" There was a touch of panic in her voice.

"What's your ETA?" a man asked.

"Three minutes."

"Okay. Open the IV fluids wide open, both IVs ...."

As the doctor's orders continued, I stopped listening because I knew what they were trying to do—keep me alive for the next three minutes until I reached the hospital. There was a team waiting there to perform miracles, if they could just keep me alive a bit longer! The pain didn't matter. How I longed for the anesthesia that would come with surgery. *Lord*, I said silently. *I wish my mom didn't have dementia and that she could be here with me. She'd run her fingers through my hair, caress my face and arms, and I'd feel so much better. I know that's impossible, Lord! But if anyone ever needed a miracle ....* I opened my eyes and rolled them upward as if to say, *I GIVE UP!*

And there she was, standing behind me, all in white. Not my mother. An Angel in the form of a young woman. She had the most lovely, silky, long, straight dark hair. Her eyes were closed as she spoke quietly. I turned my head to hear what she was saying, but she spoke in only the softest of whispers. Then she bowed, lowering her upper body over mine and covering my face with her open hands, palms down. Her hands stopped about two inches from my face and her face stopped about two inches above her hands. She never opened her eyes, and she never stopped her soft, tender whispering. Even though her hands were between my face and hers, I could see her entire face.

That's when I felt God's presence in the form of His beautiful messenger. He told me He had sent Her to pray for me. Instantly, a peace like I had never felt before came over me. A peace that passes all understanding! Everything else fell away—the blare of the siren, the sway of the ambulance, the flurry of activity to keep me alive. She was all I could see. Even though she had long, beautiful hair, her hair never moved out of place or touched me, nor did she touch me with her hands. She slowly moved towards her left as she turned the corner of my litter. She moved her hands away from my face and over my throat all the while continuing to whisper prayers with her eyes closed. Her hands moved to my chest over the top of my lungs. My eyes locked on her face. I was no longer struggling to breathe, but taking in long, slow delicious breaths. She never paused, moving her hands over my abdomen, my pelvis, the tops of my legs, my knees, and my calves, and suddenly I realized I was free of all pain! IT WAS GONE!

I closed my eyes. I didn't need to watch Her do Her work any longer. It was enough to know that She had interceded on my behalf, that She freed me from pain in a way that no medication had been able to do.

And then I understood. *I must be dying.*

It was time to say my own final prayer.

Lord, I think You are ready to bring me home to You. And since You've given me an easy end by taking away all my pain, I know that You will watch over and protect my husband, my children, my family, and my friends.

After that, I lost consciousness. I was unconscious when I arrived at Yale. Later, Rod told me he was able to see me and kiss me while I was lying on a litter in the hallway. The emergency room was so busy, I didn't actually have a room since I was going right into surgery anyway. He said I told him I loved him very much, but I don't remember that. I had lost a lot of blood and remained unconscious.

While I was out of it, a doctor met up with us outside the elevator. He had been called out of a surgery that was just ending to join the team already prepping for me in the operating room.

He introduced himself to Rod. "I'm Dr. James Yue. I'm a spine, trauma, and orthopedic surgeon, and I'll be part of the team performing your wife's surgery tonight."

"Nice to meet you, Dr. Yue," Rod responded. "Could you please do your best to save Kim's legs? She's a nurse and a runner and she has cared for other people all her life. She needs those legs." Tears dropped to his cheeks.

"Maybe you don't understand," Dr. Yue said with frankness but not without compassion. "I'm not even sure we can save her life. But we'll do our very best."

"Oh," Rod whispered. "Thank you." He dropped his gaze to the floor, staring blankly until the elevator doors opened, and they wheeled me in.

I went into surgery exactly five hours and fifty-five minutes after the accident. The survival rate after a catastrophic injury is extremely poor if the patient doesn't make it into surgery before the six-hour mark. I was hanging onto life with the barest of time to spare.

PART II

....

ARMY BRAT

No matter how much it hurts now,
someday you will look back and
realize your struggles changed
your life for the better.

—*Unknown*

CHAPTER 3

....

ON THE MOVE

I was born in October 1956 in Shillington, a small suburban town in southeastern Pennsylvania. I was the youngest of three children and the only girl. Kevin was two years older than me and Kenny nine years older. Kevin and I were best friends when we were kids, but Kenny always seemed so much older than us, more like an uncle or cousin than a brother. We didn't spend much time with him.

By the time Dad went back to active duty in the U.S. Army in 1959 after more than a decade off, Kenny was in junior high and wanted nothing to do with the military. Kenny wanted to stay in one place, make friends, and put down roots. Every time we moved, he grew angry and anxious with having to start over. It's not an exaggeration to say the moves traumatized him in some ways.

Maybe because we were younger and it was all we knew, Kevin and I loved the military life. We liked moving and living in all those different places, Virginia and New Jersey and Kansas and Wisconsin. I remember having a good childhood. I don't remember everything about it, but a few random memories stand out.

Even as a child I was friendly and outgoing. My mother has told me that I loved to stand in the front of our house, high above the sidewalk, on a stone wall my dad built, waiting for people to walk by so I could say hello.

One day while I waited on the wall, I held what I considered to be the most beautiful pair of earrings I'd ever seen. They were my mother's. Each one had a small pearl in the center surrounded by purple stones. There were special screws on the back, and I knew that was how Mom attached them to her ears. I had watched her put them on many times.

That day I had "borrowed" the earrings to try them out. While I sat on the rock wall, I tried to put them on my tiny earlobes. One of them slipped through my fingers, though, and dropped into a crack in the wall. I desperately tried to dig it out, but my fingers were too small.

I had to tell Mom. I was sure I'd be punished, but I knew I had to tell the truth. To my amazement, Mom took it in stride and didn't even get angry or punish me. She retrieved the earring from the rocks without much difficulty. All she said was that in the future I should ask if I wanted to use her things.

How silly that I had been worried about telling the truth. I learned two lessons that day. One, that Mom really loved me. And, two, always tell the truth. I've carried these lessons with me all my life.

✦ ✦ ✦

When Mom told us we were moving, I didn't understand what she meant. At two-and-a-half years old, I didn't know what the U.S. Army was or why we were leaving the only place I knew as home. She told me our new home would be in Fort Lee, Virginia, where my dad would now be stationed.

In Fort Lee our new house was joined up with other houses in a row. We were on one end. The houses all looked the same, except we had a big playground in our back yard. I felt as if I was the luckiest little girl ever! Mom also took me across the street and through the woods to a much larger playground that had a real military tank, a half-track, and the more usual playground equipment like swings and slides. Every day on the playground I met new children with new names and faces to remember.

My brother Kevin attended school, but I wasn't old enough. Because I was so eager and curious, though, Mom taught me how to read from Kevin's books. I was a sponge, very observant, and I learned quickly and had a good memory.

Kevin and I were very different. He was careful and a saver, and I was not. I was impulsive and spontaneous. I wanted to do everything *right now*. I colored every picture in my coloring book all in a rush, but he colored his book one page at a time. (I admit that sometimes when I finished my book, I tore pages out of his to color.) When we got a box of candy, I ate mine quickly, while he saved his for later. I used one of mom's pins to make a little hole in the bottom of the candy to make sure it was one I liked. If it wasn't, I switched it out with one I liked from Kevin's box. Then when I emptied my box, I started in on Kevin's bottom layer. I was still so young I really thought he wouldn't notice and wouldn't know who was eating his candy. He was pretty good about it though, and never got too angry.

One day Dad came home for lunch and afterwards as he left, I walked him out to his car. I paid special attention when he dropped an Aspergum Chicklet on the ground. He retrieved it and placed it in his mouth. He explained that he had a headache and that piece of gum was a special medicine. Later that afternoon, I found a piece of chewing gum on the ground and put it in my mouth. When I returned home, Mom said, "Where did you get that gum?"

"I found it, just like Dad!"

It took her a second to figure out what I meant. "Oh, honey! Yuck! Don't pick up anything and put it in your mouth! You'll get sick."

Mom always corrected me gently. I was never afraid when she did so. She had a way about her of making you feel good. She was a housewife, always working around the house, and she hummed or sang as she did.

One day while watching her clean I said, "You seem to be such a happy person."

She smiled. "I am a happy person. How did you know?"

"Because you always hum or sing while you work." I thought for a bit, then I asked, "Mom, do you love me?"

She stopped what she was doing. "Of course I love you. Why would you ask that?"

"I just don't remember you telling me." Well, I knew she probably had, but I wanted to hear it again.

"I do love you," she said. "And I want you to remember that forever and ever."

✦ ✦ ✦

We lived in Fort Lee until I was six years old.

My Dad's next posting was South Korea, where he was assigned to the First Army Headquarters along the Demilitarized Zone. What he did there was classified, so we never learned what it was. He stayed there for about a year.

Since we couldn't move to South Korea with Dad, Mom moved us back to Shillington for the duration. She found a ranch house in a new development named West Hills, and enrolled us in school.

I hadn't gone to kindergarten, but I was almost seven and a fluent reader, so I was placed in first grade. On one of my first days, Mrs. Hartsall had me read from one of the primary readers, which I did without missing a word. She was convinced I had memorized the pages, so she found another book and had me read that one too. She was finally convinced I was truly reading. After that, the top reading group was called Kim's Reading Group.

I loved school, and was very good in all subjects. The teachers said that I was the most fluent child in first grade. I've always taken pride in that.

One day while we were at recess, a lady ran out on the front porch of the beauty shop next to the school, and screamed, "The President's been shot!"

Recess ended immediately. I remember the profound sadness as we all watched the news about President Kennedy's assassination over the next few days. Mom seemed especially sad. I heard her tell my aunt that she worried about Dad. I was too young to understand why, but old enough to understand how worried she was.

Then one day Mom told us that Dad was coming home to a new assignment.

"Where are we moving next?" I asked. I was learning that every time Dad changed posts, we moved to a new home.

"Fort Riley, Kansas," she said.

"You mean where Dorothy and Toto live?"

"I guess so," she giggled.

"Oh, Mom I can't wait to see what Kansas is like! Where's our globe? I want to see where Kansas is and all of the states we'll drive through to get there."

Once I found the globe, I spun it a few times to watch it twirl before I stopped it and searched for Kansas. "I found it," I said, pressing my finger on the rectangle almost directly in the middle of the United States. Mom was looking over my shoulder. "Wow, that's really far from here!" I said. "It's going to take us a long time to get there, Mom."

"Probably two days."

"Does that mean we'll stay in a motel?"

"We'll have to wait and see."

With the globe in my hands, I ran out of the room and hollered for Kevin. "Kevin, you're not going to believe where we're moving next. I found it on the globe."

We met up in the living room and together looked at Kansas on the globe. We both were excited. "Wouldn't it be fun to meet Dorothy and Toto when we get there? I DO NOT want to see that nasty wicked witch, though!"

"Me neither," Kevin said, ever the good sport.

"I'm going to go tell Susanne and Maryann." I ran out the front door to tell my friends.

+ + +

By the time the school year ended, Dad was home from Korea. We each packed a small suitcase, and once our furniture was packed and loaded into the moving van, we headed West. I had never been on a car ride that long, and many times over the next few days I asked the same question, "Are we there yet?" I'm sure I drove my parents crazy. It was very hot outside and the only air conditioning we had was what came through our open windows. The further west we traveled, the hotter it became.

When we finally arrived at Fort Riley, Kansas, one of the first things I saw was a huge bison. I thought, *WOW a state that has Dorothy, Toto, bison, and me!*

The base itself was dotted with big, beautiful stone houses reserved for generals. Why couldn't my daddy be a general? He was Chief Warrant Officer, a pretty high rank in between enlisted men and commissioned officers, but not high enough for a mansion. He was in charge of all the supplies ordered for the base.

It was on that base I first developed a sense of patriotism. Every day at five sharp "Retreat" and "To the Color" were played on loud-speakers over the entire base. Cars stopped and every military person got out and saluted for the length of the two songs. When they were over, everyone got back into their cars and continued on.

We found a single-family home to lease in Junction City, a short distance south of the military base. It was a quiet suburban town within walking distance of school and a small convenience store. Kansas State University was also nearby. Our older brother Ken was going to college there. We lived next door to our landlord Mr. and Mrs. Ried, a very nice, elderly couple.

I started second grade in Miss Barkman's class at Franklin Elementary School. Miss Barkman scared me from the second my eyes met hers. She was an older woman (at least to me) and big, and she wore grannie dresses that weren't quite long enough to cover her rather large legs. Our first day of school, she laid into several students, and I thought she was mean. To my surprise, though, she took a liking to me. I became Miss Barkman's pet!

Every day she'd ask me to walk out to her car to get the large, heavy wicker picnic basket that contained her lunch. I'd pick another classmate to walk with me. One day I chose Margaret, my best friend from Germany.

I often wondered what was in that basket; it was so heavy. Once we had the basket, I said to Margaret, "Let's take a peek."

Margaret giggled. "Okay." We hid behind the stairwell, and I gently lifted the red and white gingham napkin. All we saw were several needles and syringes, which sat on the top of everything else. I swallowed hard as my eyes met Margaret's. "She eats NEEDLES for lunch!" I replaced the napkin, and smoothed it out. Margaret and I barely made a sound when we re-entered the classroom and took our seats. We were quiet for the rest of the day, but when we looked at each other, we rolled our eyes and giggled. Now that I'm an adult, I realize Miss Barkman was probably diabetic, but to second-grade me this was proof that Miss Barkman was a bizarre creature I didn't want to mess with.

One other thing stuck with me from Miss Barkman's class. Each student was required to pay a small amount of money towards the cost of our schoolbooks. Most students took care of it right away, but one student, Karen, still hadn't paid months into the school year. Every morning without fail Miss Barkman asked if her mom had sent the money. Every day the answer was "No, Miss Barkman." I had seen the rundown house Karen and her many brothers and sisters lived in, and I figured her parents might not have the money to spare. Why didn't Miss Barkman realize that?

This morning's interrogation went on for a long time. On one such morning deep into the fall, Miss Barkman asked Karen, "Did your mom give you the money for your books today?"

Karen's reply was different that day. "No. Miss Barkman. But my mommy told me to tell you to kiss her ass, we're moving!"

The room fell silent. We were too afraid to move or breathe. If Miss Barkman ate needles for lunch, none of us would live to make it home that day.

But Miss Barkman did the most surprising thing of all—nothing. She looked at Karen, then the rest of us, and shrugged, as if to say, "Why bother?"

When I got home from school, I couldn't wait to tell Mom. I wasn't sure how Mom would take it, though. Karen had been disrespectful and used a bad word besides. When I told her the story, though, she laughed long and hard. When she went quiet, she said, "You're going to have to tell your daddy that one." Dad thought it was the funniest thing he heard in a long time as well.

It became a family gag. Whenever things got a little slow at the dinner table or a family gathering, either Mom or Dad would tell me to tell the story again. We laughed hysterically every time.

One day my brother and I were playing on the front porch when a lizard darted across the concrete and disappeared into a tiny hole. I jumped. He scared me, this pre-historic looking creature. I had never seen a lizard before. *He must live under the porch*, I thought. *Will he come after me at night?* After a while, curiosity took over. I thought, *Are there a lot of lizards in Kansas? How did it get here? Does he have a mom, too? I wonder how ancient he is.* Like many children, I had a zillion questions, but I mostly kept them to myself. *Where did the little lizard really live? Was he hungry? What does he eat? What would he feel like if I ever got the chance to hold him? Was he slimy or cold or hot? Would my heart ever stop pounding when he surprised me?*

Silently I'd wait in my chair, wondering if he would come out. Sometimes he did, and sometimes he didn't. If he didn't, I soon lost interest and ran off to play. When he did come out, I watched him carefully. Sometimes I would chase him, and he would scurry away and hide. I never did catch him or touch him; he was always faster than me. But my heart did eventually stop pounding when I paused to watch him, and one day I realized I wasn't afraid of the lizard anymore. He was cute and mysterious, a small delicate creature. I didn't need to catch him. Watching him was enough.

Why do I remember that lizard so vividly? I don't really know. I was only a child, trying to figure out my world. That lizard and I shared something fundamental, two creatures in the world, separate but together.

I remember Kansas as playtime. My brother and I and the neighborhood kids played outside until well after dark and our moms called us in for the night. It was a safe warm place with a night sky sprinkled with more stars than I had ever seen before. Katydids sang their night songs, then left their shells on the trees when their songs were done. Somedays our moms would walk us to a large fountain several blocks from home and let us splash around to cool off. Eventually, my parents bought a large, round swimming pool for our backyard, and everyone enjoyed coming over to play and swim. We loved our playtime and hated those rainy days we were stuck inside.

Sometimes Kevin and I played outside with Dad's gas masks. He had an older one from World War II, my brother's favorite, and a newer one I wore. I wonder what our neighbors thought when they saw us playing hide-and-seek in our gas masks running between yards and in the back alley like creatures from outer space. We also played with Dad's machete, hacking at the tree trunks in our yard. I don't think our parents knew about that game. They surely would have put a stop to it.

In our world, even cleaning could be fun. My mother put my brother and me on the enclosed back porch with mops and a bucket of water. We refilled the bucket over and over, dumped it out, then slapped the water this way and that with the mop and eventually out the open door. We did this for hours.

One day my brother invented another game our parents didn't know about. With silver tape, he attached the long nails he found in Dad's toolbox to each one of his fingers, and he became a superhero! My friend and I wanted to be superheroes, too, but my hypercompetitive brother said we could only have five nails. We went along with him for a while, then when no one was watching, I darted onto the porch. I was all for fairness and equality. I taped five other nails in place, and I took five more for my friend. I pushed open the door to run outside, but there he was, my brother, always one step ahead of me! We were both running fast and slammed into each other. I saw stars and then I saw blood gushing from his mouth. We both yelled.

I was scared. *Was I in trouble? How could I help him? What should I do? Mom and Dad are going to kill us!* All these thoughts went through my mind as we lay there calling for help. Mom heard us and ran out with a dish towel that she clamped to his mouth. She got him to the hospital—I don't remember how. He had practically bitten his tongue off, but the doctors managed to stitch it up, and in a few weeks the stitches melted away and Kevin could eat solid food again.

Of course our parents didn't kill us, but they did give us a stern talking to about playing safely and paying attention when we were running around the yard. I was sorry Kevin got hurt, but I wasn't sorry I stood up for myself. I learned early in life that if you wanted things to be fair, you had to fight for them.

Sometimes Mom would take a break from her housework to join us in a game of cards. My brother was very competitive, and I usually lost except when Mom cheated so I could win. Boy, did that make my brother mad. He thought winning was everything. I enjoyed winning every once in a while, but if he lost, he'd throw his cards on the table, call me a baby, and run from the room. It was never about the winning for me, more about the fun of playing together. But that's not how he saw it. He wanted to win at all costs, creating a kind of one-sided sibling rivalry, which I tried to ignore. It took its toll, though. I often felt I was fighting for some unnamed prize according to rules no one ever told me. I've always tried to teach my kids to avoid this kind of fruitless sibling rivalry, but I'm not sure they understood. It was something they had to learn for themselves.

In many ways, my childhood was filled with all kinds of uncomplicated wonders, but I was growing older and fears and anxieties crept in. I knew my father loved us, but he wasn't openly affectionate, and when he didn't think anyone was watching, I'd see him sink into himself as if he was trying to disappear. Mom was the best mom ever, better than any mom on TV, loving and caring and never raising her hand or voice to us. But then I'd see her watching Dad with a helpless sadness I couldn't explain.

And then there were the letters.

I was in the storm cellar with Mom, a cool and spooky place. You entered the cellar from the back of the house by opening two wooden doors that lay on its frame at an angle to the ground like a huge wedge of cake. It was like Dorothy's house in the movie. Then you walked down several concrete steps to the dirt floor, which always smelled of must and dust. Mom was going through some of our moving boxes when she discovered a secret hiding place covered by a dirty piece of wood. What's not cool about a secret hiding place?

She pulled out a box that had collapsed in on itself, and from the box she took out a bundle of envelopes. She thumbed through the envelopes, then pulled out a letter, read a few lines, turned it over to check the signature, then burst into tears. They were written to Mr. Ried, she explained, during World War II, but not by Mrs. Ried. "Mrs. Ried should never find these letters," she said between sobs. "They were already married during the war."

Mom gathered up the letters, marched up the cellar stairs, stuffed them into our burning can, then struck a match and dropped it in among the papers. She occasionally stirred the fire with a stick and watched sadly until the letters were ash.

I didn't get it at the time. It was just a bunch of letters, and not even Dad's. But as I grew older, the pieces fell into place, and I wondered what sadness of her own Mom was projecting on those long-hidden, illicit love letters from World War II.

With all these fragmented glimpses into the world of adults, that summer was the first time in my life I remember being afraid without knowing why.

When we first moved to Kansas, the shriek of the night train whistle startled me awake. But after a while, I played so hard during the day that most nights I fell asleep without a problem. The whistle turned into a lullaby and the sound of the trains gave me a sense of peace that helped me fall asleep. To this day, when I see the trains of the Union Pacific Railroad, I smile.

Other nights I couldn't fall asleep at all, that nameless fear rattling around in my head and keeping me up. I lay awake for hours, my eyes gritty, watching the reflections on the walls and ceiling, the lights flickering, my heart pounding hard. I tried to think myself asleep. *Don't be afraid, the house is safe. You are safe. Everyone is safe. Fall asleep. Fall asleep. Fall asleep.* Sometimes I felt as if I never slept, but I usually did, eventually, though I'd wake up in the morning buzzing with exhaustion.

Soon I'd have actual cause to worry.

CHAPTER 4

DAD GOES TO VIETNAM

It was the summer of 1965. Dad came home with the news that Grandma Baur (his mother) was coming to visit the entire summer. About ten years after Grandpa Baur died (he died so young that even Mom never met him), Grandma Baur sold the house in Shillington and split time with her children after that, moving from house to house every two or three months. That summer it was our turn.

We had mixed feelings about this news. We loved Grandma Baur, of course, but today we'd say she had problems with boundaries. She snooped through our drawers when no one was home, and as I grew older, I felt this invasion of privacy more deeply, as did Mom, who felt Grandma was always trying to show her up in her own house. In junior high, I put a piece of paper in each drawer that read: *I caught you, so stop looking in my drawers*. It was a nice try, but had no real effect. Dad and Kevin didn't seem to mind as much.

Less than a week later we drove to the airport in Kansas City to pick her up. We were all looking forward to introducing her to another fun Kansas summer. Not long after Grandma arrived, though, Dad came home with a serious look on his face. He had new orders.

Instead of spending another summer in Kansas, we were headed to Wisconsin, where Dad was assigned for the summer to Fort McCoy in the Northern part of the state. His job was to get the Fifth Army supplied and ready for a huge campaign that was coming in a faraway country called Vietnam.

Space was limited in our green Chevy sedan. Kevin and I shared a suitcase. Ken was staying in Kansas in his fraternity house. We packed that green Chevy until nothing else could possibly fit. Mom and Dad had to sit on the trunk lid to get it closed.

Dad drove, Mom rode shotgun, and I sat between them. Kevin and Grandma were in the back seat, separated by suitcases stacked to the ceiling. We didn't have seatbelts and we didn't have air conditioning, but we had big windows and air vents, which only seemed to blast dust particles into my eyes.

Mom and Dad found a furnished place on a large dairy farm just outside of Tomah, Wisconsin. Mr. and Mrs. Sites had a second-floor apartment, a perfect summer rental.

As a military kid, I was used to sudden moves, and even enjoyed new names and faces. Mr. and Mrs. Sites were wonderful people and they loved showing my brother and me around their farm. Our apartment wasn't air conditioned, but with the crisp night air in that part of Wisconsin, we didn't really need it. After a while even the manure smelled oddly familiar, reminding me of our home in Pennsylvania.

Even though my brother and I loved to swim, we didn't go swimming once that summer. The water was too cold! The one day Mom dropped us off at the community swimming pool, we dipped our feet in the water and said, "Nope, can't do it." We still had fun as a family, though. We traveled around Wisconsin sampling—what else?—delicious cheeses.

We had our adventures as well. One day, Mrs. Sites knocked on our apartment door to tell us that Dad was on the phone, that the car had broken down, and that he needed the checkbook to pay for repairs. He told Mom he would wait in a bar in the town of Tomah.

That was quite a distance from us, but Mom said, "Don't worry, we'll get there."

Mr. Sites was away for the day, so we couldn't hitch a ride with him. There was only one thing left to do. Mom, Kevin, and I left Grandma in the apartment to snoop to her heart's content and headed out on foot. It seemed as if it would take us forever to get there, with the huge farms and the farm roads that went on and on. After we walked for what *I* thought was forever, a car passed us, then slowed down and pulled over. It was no doubt unusual to see a mother and her two children walking on the side of that long stretch of country road. "Can I give you a ride?" the man in the car asked politely.

My mother said, "Sure, we need a ride to Tomah. My husband's car broke down."

"I'd be happy to take you into town," the man said. "Tomah is quite a ways on foot." He got out to help us with the car door.

At some point when we were riding in the man's car, I said loudly to my mother, "You told us to never take rides with strangers. Why are we in this car?" I always remembered what Mom told me.

She explained that he was a kind man and that she was with us and this time it was okay.

He took us exactly where we needed to be, and we met up with Dad. We waited in the bar until the repairs were finished, since it was the only place with air conditioning, or so Dad said. That must have been the same reason we stopped at so many bars on our way from Kansas to Wisconsin. We'd get something to eat, Dad would have a drink or two, then we'd get back on the road. I thought nothing of it. Didn't all fathers need a drink at regular intervals to keep going?

The summer in Wisconsin ended abruptly when Dad was ordered back to Kansas. He got one day's notice for all of us and our possessions to head back to Kansas in the green Chevy. Those orders must have been very important.

We had moved out of our house in Kansas and all our furniture was in storage. Mom, who was always in charge of our moves, found a furnished apartment in Manhattan, Kansas, on the third floor of a new apartment complex called the Wild Cat Creek Apartments. Grandma Baur was still with us, which made the apartment cramped.

It was my first time living in an apartment. I didn't care for the Formica table and counter tops or the flimsy sofa with four-inch cushions through which you could feel a hard sheet of plywood against your bottom. We usually just sat on the floor to watch TV. The good news was that there was more than one swimming pool in the complex, and a gigantic dumpster my brother and I climbed into to rummage around. Another one of our games Mom didn't know about. We found tumbleweeds in the fields as well as our first piece of petrified wood. You have to hand it to me and my brother. We always knew how to keep busy.

Early in the fall of 1965, my father learned that the First Infantry Division—his division, also known as the Big Red One because of their red shoulder patches—was going to Vietnam. The First Division was a legendary combat infantry division, with roots in World War I, and Dad was proud to be part of it.[1] There is a 1980 movie called *The Big Red One* set in World War II.

Once Dad was deployed, Grandma Baur moved in with Uncle Stewart (Stut) and Aunt Gerry, who lived in York, Pennsylvania.

Vietnam was different for Mom, more difficult, and it wasn't until I grew older that I understood why. Dad had been in Korea for a year, but there wasn't a war in Korea at the time, and he returned safely. But Vietnam was—Vietnam, an actual shooting war (though it was never officially declared), and U.S. involvement was ramping up. My Dad was part of that, and Mom cried every day from worry. She tried to hide it from us, but she couldn't, and her worry made us worry. We all lived with a heightened sense of dread. Every night we watched Walter Cronkite recap the war, and every night Mom cried herself to sleep. Mom and Dad exchanged letters daily. She thought it was important to help Dad keep that connection to home, and it gave her something to do to pass the time.

After a while, Mom couldn't take it anymore. Although school was going well for my brother and me in the new open-concept school we attended, one day Mom told us we were headed back to my grandparents' farm in Pennsylvania until Dad returned. She thought we'd have more support there and we could get to know our cousins. More importantly, though, Mom would have her parents and sister Shirley to turn to.

Mom was never good with driving for any length of time. I have no idea how she managed this trip alone with a nine-year-old and an eleven-year-old. I don't know how many days it took, or where we spent the nights. All I know is that suddenly things looked familiar and we were in Gouglersville, Pennsylvania. I started school the next day a mile away from my grandparents' farm. The school sat atop a hill next to the church we attended. Mrs. Drysbock was my teacher, and her husband was our pastor. It was a nice little farming community.

When we weren't in school, Kevin and I did what we did best—explored our grandparents' farm and got to know our cousins, especially Shirley's two older sons, Jeff and Greg. Grandpa and Grandma had several cows, pigs, chickens, and roosters, numerous barn cats, and a dog. There was a meadow that was electrically fenced for the cows and a stream that ran through the meadow. They grew corn and hay in large fields and Grandma kept a huge vegetable garden. She made jam and canned and froze her fruits and vegetables. She baked bread and made a fresh dessert every day.

The barn had two-stories, a cold cellar, and several outbuildings. One of the first things we did was build a fort in the haystack on the second floor. Our fort was up so high we could touch the massive wooden rafters. We were also able to peep out the knotholes in the walls to see who was calling us. We got out of the fort by climbing down the ladder or jumping into the pile of hay in the hay wagon. Then we'd take a long slide down the hay hole grandfather used to slide the bales of hay to the cattle on the first floor. We found this easier to do once we moved the pitchfork.

The chicken coop also tempted us. Inside the air was thick with a mixture of dust, feathers, and stench. Each chicken had its own place to sit, and my grandma reached underneath the chickens to take the eggs when she found one. We weren't brave enough to check for eggs. Some were spotted with poop! Instead, we had the great idea of running through the chicken house screaming and hollering until the chickens were in a tizzy, flying around the chicken house, smacking into the walls and each other. When Grandma saw what we were doing, she chased us out and told us to find another place to play. She never found out about the chicken Kenny and Gale parachuted from the second story of the barn. That poor chicken didn't lay eggs for a week.

I liked watching Grandma milk the cows in the late afternoon after she brought them back to the barn from the meadow. The stray cats she had adopted always knew when to show up to sample the milk before she brought it inside. She'd put some of the milk into her wooden butter churn, and I'd help her make fresh butter. Then we chilled the rest.

I loved to watch all the things my grandma did. She was a stocky woman and always wore a dress with a full apron over the top. When she baked and cooked, she used every part of every item of her garden. She never used a recipe, yet everything always tasted delicious. I asked her how she did that, and she told me that she judged ingredients based on consistency rather than amount. She made the best strawberry rhubarb pie, which I loved. Mom's favorite was her pumpkin pie. She also made donuts from scratch, filling her entire table while they cooled. If anyone wanted one of her recipes, they had to watch her make the dish and do their best to estimate the amounts she used. She kept it all in her head.

Grandma liked candy as much as I did, and she kept it hidden in jars around the farmhouse, though when I asked, she always told me where I could find some. She bought the candy at the Green Dragon, the best Amish market in Lancaster County, Pennsylvania. Sometimes I went with her and watched her pick out what she wanted in small quantities—a quarter-pound of this, a half-pound of that, ten or fifteen different kinds of candies in little white bags we carried home.

For church, she kept spearmint leaves and licorice chips in her purse. If I pretended I had a tickle in my throat, she'd quietly open her purse and pass me one. I knew the perfect noise to make.

I thought she was the best grandma ever, a saint really. I never remember her yelling, even that day we chased her chickens. All she said was, "Okay kids, that's not what we do on the farm." We knew that we had to listen to her, since Grandpa was behind her. We didn't want him to find out we were doing something wrong. The consequences were much more severe, sometimes harsh yelling, sometimes spankings.

When my cousins came to the farm, we'd play hide and seek after dark. We played until we heard THE WOOD CHOPPER, who in our vivid childhood imaginations was a monster out of a horror movie. The sound of him chopping from somewhere deep in the woods scared us so much we ran inside. Grandpa loved to tell tales about how the woodchopper hid gold in the woods and how he and others gone searching for the woodchopper, but no one ever found him or the gold. But if you were brave enough to follow the sound of his chopping after dark ... you might get lucky.

When it snowed, everyone showed up at the farm with their sleds. We walked a quarter mile to the top of the highest hill and made a long train. Each child held onto the sled in front of them and hooked their feet into the sled behind them. When everyone was linked, we pushed off down the hill, our screams and laughter loud in the cold air. We crashed long before we reached the end of the run. Then we rushed to the top to do it again and again all day long.

Every day was a new adventure. We made a tree swing from heavy-duty rope and an old tire, and we passed hours swinging. We found a sour cherry tree that produced delicious cherries. We sucked on honeysuckle to taste the sweet nectar and chewed on birch root, which gives root beer its flavor. At dusk we caught lightning bugs and put them in jars with holes punched in the lids.

Mom was the second of the eleven children born on the farm, all delivered at home. Mom thought Grandma was a saint too. She remembered only one time when her mom was grouchy. On that occasion, in the middle of the night, Mom heard a newborn crying. She realized many years later that her mother must have been in labor that night. Farm women are tough as leather, and Grandma was no exception. I thank the Lord every day that she passed on some of her toughness to me.

Kevin and I thought we had died and gone to kid heaven, but Mom didn't like the way Grandpa disciplined us. Mom was advanced for her time. She disciplined us with words and timeouts. She was too loving to imagine hurting any of God's creatures, let alone her own children. She didn't approve of yelling and spanking, and Grandpa was a spare-the-rod-spoil-the-child kind of disciplinarian. Perhaps it was a flash-back to her childhood. Whatever the case, once school was over, Mom hauled us back to Kansas.

We arrived in Kansas after a tornado had passed through Manhattan. One whole wall of bricks was torn off the apartment building we had lived in. When I searched through the debris, as I liked to do, I found a brick impaled by blade of wheat. On one side of the brick, you could see the kernel, and on the other side you could see the stem. How did that happen? The power of that tornado must have been incredible to turn a flexible strand of wheat into a dangerous projectile with enough force to pierce a brick! I couldn't grasp it then, and I still can't grasp it.

This was the summer of 1966, and though we were no longer on the farm, Mom tried her best to keep us entertained. We swam every day in one of the apartment swimming pools, and Mom took us to the twenty-five cent movies on the Army base. On our way home we stopped for an ice cream sundae or a banana split. We saw my older brother from time to time when he wasn't busy at college.

But Dad was still in Vietnam, and that put a pall over everything we did that summer.

CHAPTER 5

....

MUSTERED OUT

I remember the day Mom told us Dad was coming home from Vietnam. I can still remember what Mom wore when we picked him up. She looked so beautiful in her pink and white gingham skirt and blouse pulled together with a small green belt with green balls at each end. (I still have that outfit. It reminds me of that day.) My dad's hair was shorter than I had ever seen it, practically shaved. He said it was because it was so hot in Vietnam.

We went to the base to pick him up. I remember him walking down the steps of the bus and Mom running to hug and kiss him just like in the movies. Kevin and I followed her lead, and he hugged and kissed us too. We picked up Kenny from Kansas State, and Mom made us all dinner—the first full family dinner in a year. After dinner, Kevin and I played outside for a few hours, while my parents celebrated with a bottle of wine on our apartment deck. Once the wine was finished, Mom told us to go to bed, and then, well, I assume Mom and Dad got reacquainted.

Dad drank a lot more after he returned from Vietnam, and he became two different people. When he wasn't drinking (or drinking less), he was the nice person I knew before he left, asking me questions about my day or complimenting a picture I had colored. When he was drinking, though, he said and did bizarre things, ranting about people coming after us and picking fights with Mom. Although my brother didn't seem to care, their fighting always upset me. When they fought, my world threatened to come apart. That's when I turned into Little Mom, acting the adult to get them to stop. Sometimes I screamed louder than they did just so they'd hear me. If that didn't work, I jumped up and down on the bed until they stopped arguing. None of us could figure out what was going on in Dad's head and why he came home from Vietnam so different.

One day Dad came home with a new assignment, and just like that we moved again, this time to Fort Dix in New Jersey. I made friends immediately with Kimberly who lived on the base just two blocks from us. She was my first Black friend. We rode our bikes around the base or played outside like I had played everywhere we moved in my short life.

Kimberly had a strange habit—she ate Vaseline. She scooped it out of the jar with her index finger and plopped it in her mouth. I dry heaved the first time I saw her do that, and I always wondered why her parents let her. (As an adult, I learned that petroleum jelly is actually safe to eat, that some people used it as a laxative, but I still wonder why you would want to!)

Kevin and I soon discovered the storm sewers running under the base when we found the outlet into the small creek near our house. We grabbed our flashlights and set off to explore. We didn't have storm sewers in Kansas and certainly not on my grandparents' farm. Sometimes we turned off our flashlights in the sewers and relied on the light from the storm drains. We could barely see, but it was fun to run through the pipes in the dark screaming to hear our voices echo. Our fun ended when Mom found out where we had been playing and forbade us from going in there again.

While we lived in New Jersey, my parents had quite a few military functions to attend in the evenings. Kevin and I stayed home by ourselves. Mom bought us a Chef Boyardee pizza at the commissary, and we felt so grown up making our own dinner. I don't think Mom had as good a time on those nights as we did, though. Dad usually came home drunk, which he was doing more often. On nights he didn't go out with Mom, he went to the Officer's Club, and when he missed dinner, Mom would drag us with her to get him to come home. If he wouldn't come home for her, she told us, maybe he'd come home for his children.

We hadn't seen our grandparents since we lived with them, so they planned a trip to visit us in New Jersey for a week. They didn't leave the farm often because of the animals and the chores, but some of my aunts and uncles agreed to help in their absence.

Unfortunately, my grandfather was not an experienced driver, and he was unfamiliar with roundabouts, of which New Jersey at that time had quite a few. As my grandfather approached one roundabout in particular in his big, white Cadillac, he thought he had the right of way and that the car approaching from the other direction would yield. Grandpa continued into the circle without stopping, and hit the other car head on. The cars had no seat belts. Grandma's face broke through the windshield, and Grandpa took the force of the steering wheel to his chest. The real tragedy was that a child in the other car died in the crash.

Mom and Dad rushed to the hospital where my grandparents had been admitted. When Mom saw Grandma, she fainted. Grandma had so many lacerations from the glass shards in her face that she was unrecognizable. She went into surgery that night and received over one hundred stitches. She remained in the hospital for quite a while to heal.

Grandpa was discharged the next day, but he was extremely upset and cried throughout the day, saying he'd never forgive himself. He had killed a child and severely injured his wife. He vowed never to drive again.

Several weeks later when Grandma finally came home from the hospital, I was shocked how scarred her face was, but she was alive and that was what was important. My grandparents remained with us for several weeks while Grandma recuperated, and then one Saturday my uncle arrived and took them home to their farm. I don't think my grandparents ever quite fully recovered from that tragedy. Grandpa didn't drive a car again for many, many years and only did so once his children encouraged him to drive again to gain more freedom. Together, my grandparents continued to care for the animals and the crops in their fields until their deaths, Grandma from Leukemia in 1982, and Grandpa two years later after a heart attack.

✦ ✦ ✦

Before the school year ended my dad came home with more exciting news: we were moving again, but this time to Panama, somewhere near the famous Canal. I was so excited about this move—I had never been out of the country before! Dad seemed excited as well. I think he was bored with Fort Dix.

He told Mom he had to pass a physical exam, blood work, and an EKG before the assignment was confirmed, but he figured that would be a piece of cake. The appointments were spread out throughout the week. One day he had blood work done early in the morning. A day later he had an EKG, and then underwent a full physical examination. Early the next week, he would meet with a medical panel to discuss the results, and then he'd be confirmed.

He had a smile on his face all that week. He hadn't been this happy since he returned from Vietnam. We all had our fingers crossed the day of the medical panel meeting, but he told us we had nothing to worry about. I couldn't concentrate that day at school, and when classes were finally over, I met up with Kevin and we rushed home to hear the results.

The wretched look on Mom's face told us everything. He had failed the exam. He had called Mom as soon as he found out that afternoon, but hadn't given her any other details or where he might be assigned instead.

Mom had made chicken pot pie for dinner, my favorite. I couldn't wait for Dad to get home so we could all have dinner together. We waited and waited and waited, but no Dad. Finally Mom said, "Let's eat. Maybe he had to meet with his boss after work."

Hours after we had eaten we still hadn't heard from Dad, and Mom grew worried. Around nine, she called the Officer's Club. Instead of being angry when she talked to him, she kept telling him it was all going to be okay. When she hung up, she called my brother and me to her and explained that we were no longer going to Panama.

"Then where are we moving next?" I asked.

"I don't know," she sighed. "Now it's time for bed. Maybe we'll know more in the morning."

I saw Dad in the morning before he left. He was deep in thought, distant and sad, his smile gone. He made no jokes that morning. I had to remind him to kiss me goodbye.

Every day after that I watched him drag himself home from work. He barely spoke a word to us. He just stared into the air with a blank expression. When I talked to him, he didn't hear me even though I was just a few feet away. I wanted to hug him and tell him I loved him, but even that didn't seem to matter anymore.

Then our world spun even further out of orbit when Dad announced he would be leaving the military altogether. We would finish the school year, which was almost over, then pack up and return to Pennsylvania. The U.S. Army no longer wanted him—his health was too much of a risk. He had had a heart attack while he was in Vietnam, a silent one he never even knew about. He would receive an honorable discharge and one hundred percent disability.

Dad was devastated. His career—his life—had been taken from him literally overnight. He was only forty-four and felt as if he was in the prime of his life with much more to give to his country.

The next month dragged by. It was painful to watch my dad grieve the loss of his career. It was like watching him slowly die, piece by piece. I was just a child, so I had to follow Mom's guidance. Mom had to be strong for Dad, and she always was. The only ones excited about this move were our family members back in Pennsylvania.

The day the Allied Moving Van showed up, I said goodbye to my friends, as I had so many times before. We stayed in a motel overnight. Mom always insisted on cleaning the house one last time after the furniture was removed. The military did a white glove inspection after you left the house, and she always wanted the best possible score.

When we left the base that day, I realized that would be the last time anyone would salute my father. The life he had known for twenty-five years was over.

+ + +

My father was nineteen years old when the United States entered World War II. He enlisted in the Army immediately and was sent to basic training in Spartanburg, South Carolina. Just before his deployment, he spiked a high fever and developed a skin rash that covered his entire body. He went into a military hospital and his platoon was deployed without him. The platoon left the United States by ship heading towards the Artic Ocean. Once there, a German submarine torpedoed and sank the ship in the icy sea. Every man in Dad's platoon died. He was devastated with grief and survivor's guilt. He had trained with these men, ate with them, lived with them, and planned to go into battle with them. Why had he survived?

Once released from the hospital, my father joined the 338th Brigade, going first into North Africa and eventually into Italy. The 338th was among the forces who fought on the Gothic Line, Germany's last line of defense in the Apennine Mountains and fortified with thousands of machine gun nests, bunkers, and artillery posts. The battle was the biggest in Italy, involving upwards of 1.2 million men.

Ineffective communications made things even more difficult for the allies. Their radios often failed them in the mountainous terrain. Orders became garbled, and troops were often sent to the wrong location. One time, a soldier was sent by foot to deliver a message for backup air support and to let command know where the troops were moving. On his way, he was killed and the message was never delivered. Many more men perished.

The way Dad tells it, they fought for six full days with extremely high fatalities. Those who survived, like my dad, were changed forever by the horror of battle—the din of artillery and small arms fire, the screams of the dying and the wounded, men spouting blood and losing arms and legs, their own feelings of panic, fear, and helplessness. It was truly a living hell.

At one point, my dad dug a foxhole, but was called to a lookout post before he could use it. When he returned, he saw the foxhole had been hit by mortar fire. He didn't want to use it after that, so another soldier claimed it, telling Dad, "Did you ever hear the saying that lightning never strikes twice?" Dad nodded. "That's why I'm going to be safe here!"

Despite his exhaustion, Dad dug another foxhole. During a heavy bombardment, the soldiers retreated to the safety of their foxholes. When the firing let up, the soldiers emerged to assess the damage and assist the wounded. Dad checked out his old foxhole. It was gone, obliterated by another round of mortar fire, and the young soldier confident in his safety was dead. Once again, my father had survived. He was too busy fighting a war to process it then, but the shock, guilt, and sadness from that battle stayed buried within him for quite some time.

He stayed in Italy for four years and left the army after the war and his time at the University of Florence to own and run a plumbing business, which is what he was doing during the actual Korean war in the 1950s. He remained in the reserves during that time. It wasn't until after he rejoined the Army in 1959 that he was assigned a tour of duty in South Korea. He was there during the Cuban Missile Crisis and when President John F. Kennedy was shot and killed in Dallas.

Dad often told me that Vietnam was the worst of his deployments because it was so messy, with no clear battle lines, and because the South Vietnamese allies looked a lot like the North Vietnamese enemies, they often didn't know who they were fighting. During the day women and children stood outside the fence begging for food, chewing gum, and cigarettes. After dark, some of these same people shot at the U.S. soldiers.

Dad was a supply officer, a role that kept him very busy. He ordered and oversaw the food and supplies for the entire base. He often had to travel by helicopter into Saigon and other destinations to procure those supplies. This was quite dangerous, but he did it because he thought his men deserved the best dinners he could round up. Any meal could have been their last.

In the helicopter, the large doors on either side were always open for the gunners and the extreme jungle heat. Shots from the ground forces whizzed past the open door and mortar explosions lit up the sky like lethal fireworks.

Each soldier was safely locked into position by clipping onto an overhead cable. On one mission, my father changed his mind about where he wanted to be dropped off. Because the helicopters were noisy, he had to disconnect from the overhead safety cable and move up beside the pilot to let him know. He stood up, reached for the cable and disconnected the lead. At the exact moment he took a step, the pilot banked the helicopter into a sharp right. Dad lost his balance and fell towards the open door, unable to grab anything to catch himself. Just as he was about to tumble out the door to his death, his friend grabbed him by his loose shirt and pulled him back into the helicopter. From that point on, Dad said, he was grateful that the Army-issued fatigues never fit very well. And he never unhooked mid-flight again.

On patrol, the soldiers walked through thick jungles, encountering poisonous snakes, giant scorpions, giant centipedes, fire ants, and even tigers, as well as the enemy, who were difficult to track down and engage. The Vietcong had built sophisticated underground tunnel systems with hidden entrances. This allowed them to emerge from the tunnels unexpectedly, engage the Americans in a firefight, then disappear to safety. The jungle plants also posed a threat. Some of the low-hanging vines could grab a person and constrict whatever body part it touched first. Other plants and trees were toxic if touched or accidentally ingested. Eventually Agent Orange was used to clear the jungle vegetation for military operations, but that too, had long-term, devastating effects on military personnel and civilians.

Late at night rats scurried through the tents they bunked in. Many times, my father woke up to rats foraging through his tent, which he shared with a major. He quietly woke his tentmate, and from their beds, they shot the rats with their pistols.

With Dad's rank and status, he was sometimes called on to act as a liaison or chaperon for USO performers. Because she was a favorite of mine, he liked to tell the story of the time he was assigned to chaperone Anne Murray. Soon after she arrived in Vietnam, however, something happened, and she was promptly whisked away. He never did meet her. To this day, I love Anne Murray's music. After the accident, I listened to her over and over. She brought back my sanity. My dad loved her music too, one of the few things we had in common. Whenever one of her songs came on the radio, he would say, "That's our girl Kim, that's our girl!"

Dad was in Vietnam for about a year. When he received his orders to return to the States, he was literally in the jungle one day, hopped an extremely long flight home, and was back in Kansas the next. Talk about whiplash. He had no time to adjust, and his return was complicated by the growing unpopularity of the war and anti-war protests. It's no wonder my father suffered PTSD and resorted to alcohol, the only medicine he knew that would quickly numb the pain.

As hard as life was for Dad in the Army, it was about to become harder still.

+ + +

A pastor and his wife were leasing our home in Shillington, and the lease did not end until August. We stayed with my grandparents on their farm until my parents found a rental, another adventure as far as my brother and I were concerned—a mobile home in a small trailer park in the middle of Lancaster County surrounded by Amish farms. I wondered what it would be like to live near Amish children who didn't have electricity, running water, or toilets in their homes and traveled in horse drawn buggies.

It was another fun summer for my brother and me. We loved being in the country again and having endless playtime outside. We bought brown eggs from the Amish family farm down the road, which had twelve children. They also sold fresh fruit and vegetables from a small wooden stand just inside the gate. One time when my mom sent me over for eggs, it must have been bath day. On the side of their house was a big, round, steel tub filled with water. One by one, all the children climbed into the tub for their bath, using the same water. I felt sorry for the last few. By then, the water was covered in gray scum.

The girls wore long dresses, and their hair was pulled back in a ponytail, a pigtail, or braids. Sometimes they wore bonnets like their moms. The boys wore black pants, bright dress shirts and suspenders and straw hats to shade their faces. Their parents dressed the same, though the mothers typically wore an apron over their dress and always a bonnet to cover their hair. I liked to observe them in their environment, but they also checked us out whenever we went to their farm.

Friday evening was courting night in the Amish community. The young men cleaned their families' buggies, then attached a gas lantern for visibility. After dark, they picked up their dates in the buggies. I'm not sure where they went, since they weren't allowed to go to the movies. What I did know was that on their way home from wherever they had been, they had the horses plod along as slowly as possible to give them more time to hold hands and kiss.

Kevin and I sometimes played a joke on the couples. We hid in the gutter on the side of road and as the slow horses approached, we made a clicking sound with our mouths to get the horses galloping. We thought we were hilarious and laughed until our belly's hurt. Now, of course, I realize that we were just plain mean, and I'm glad no one got hurt.

The biggest mistake I made that summer was telling an annoying boy in the trailer park that I wasn't allergic to poison ivy. To prove my point, I picked several fresh poison ivy leaves and rubbed them all over my legs and arms. In less than twenty-four hours, a red, blistering, itchy rash broke out over most of my body. I was covered in calamine lotion for several weeks, while Mom told me not to scratch probably a million times.

Going back to Pennsylvania was a good move for me. I enjoyed living closer to relatives. We could go to my grandparents' farm anytime. One Saturday I was feeling adventurous, so I rode my bicycle to the farm. Once there, I called Mom to tell her where I was. She was shocked to realize that I had ridden over eight miles to get there. I promised her I'd be safe on my ride back home. I did stop at the dry dam bed, removing my sneakers before walking into the muck to see how far down I'd sink. When my bony knees almost disappeared, I plucked myself from the mud while I still could.

Dad was the only one who wasn't very happy with this move. He had a difficult time finding a job, and he drank to fill the empty days. He spent a lot of time in bars in nearby New Holland. Sometimes he went alone and stayed for hours. Other times, he took us with him. We enjoyed dinner while he enjoyed his liquid gold. He also drank at home alone or with relatives who came to play cards. When we didn't have visitors, he watched religious programs on TV at a high volume, the ones where evangelist preachers begged for money and talked about how we were all going to hell. They scared me. I was young enough to believe them. One of the good things was that Mom and

Dad were fighting less, maybe because Mom knew how hard it was for Dad to leave the Army.

I started fifth grade after Labor Day. My grades in school were always excellent. I simply loved school, both the social aspect and everything I was learning. I made friends easily and was kind to others. Outside of school, I had neighborhood friends and my cousins were always available for fun at the farm. Each summer Mom bought swimming pool memberships for my brother and me, and we swam daily, taking the shortcut through the convent property, though the nuns were not very happy about that. It was picturesque and serene and shortened the walk by fifteen minutes.

Dad found a job as a security guard in a drug store in Reading, about a ten-minute drive from Shillington. The city could be dangerous, and he was hired because the store was in a high crime area. Mom was not happy with the job, but it was the only one he could find. Mom also found work as a waitress in the tearoom of an upscale department store, Whitner's. She worked through the lunch hour, their busiest time.

Dad's behavior was getting more bizarre and less predictable, and because I was approaching junior high, more embarrassing to me. Sometimes it was the alcohol, but other times it wasn't. When frozen turkeys went on sale at the grocery store, he took me shopping with him. We loaded two shopping carts with the turkeys, twenty-five in all. At the checkout counter, the friendly clerk asked, "Ya having a party?"

"No," Dad said without smiling.

I wanted to crawl away. Who was this crazy stranger of a father?

I thought Mom was going to lose her mind when she came home from work to find twenty-five turkeys taking up all the space in our refrigerator and chest freezer. I don't remember if she cooked all those turkeys for us or gave some away. I can't imagine we ate them all.

I couldn't bring my friends to the house any more. It was tough enough dealing with adolescence without his strange behavior on top of it. And like adolescents everywhere, I stopped trying to figure him out and ignored him as much as I could.

The next two years flew by in a flash of school and friends. Then it was off to junior high in the fall.

I was so excited for junior high. Overnight, I felt much more grown up. I was disappointed at first when I entered Mr. Hoyer's homeroom and found none of my friends there or in any of my other classes. It never took me very long to make friends, though, and within days I had already made new friends, girls and boys both.

I gravitated to one girl, Jeannette, who seemed especially glamorous and cool. She wore beautiful clothing, and was even allowed to wear makeup. She taught me how to apply eye liner, eye shadow, mascara, and blush. Mom said it was okay for me to use makeup if I kept it to a minimum. I felt so pretty with this new look.

On weekends, we went to the high school football games. One parent took us to the game, and another picked us up. Sometimes we went to the movies and met up with boys, but usually the girls sat together, as did the boys. I was allowed to sleep over at my friends' houses if Mom knew where I was and what we would be doing. I always had to call Mom to check in. I never invited girls to sleep over at my house. It was too risky, with Dad the way he was. Everyone loved Mom, but Dad intimidated my friends with his size, presence, and silence, unless he was drinking. Then they thought he was funny, but he wasn't funny to me.

My brother Kevin and I seldom did anything together anymore. We each had our own friends. Even at home we seldom spoke, both of us in the throes of adolescence. When we did, it was usually to argue. I stayed in my bedroom much of the time I was in the house.

Mom was the only one I could talk to at home, and although we were close, I felt like I fit in better at the homes of my friends. I felt loved, accepted, and welcomed. I was always having fun and was the life of any sleepover or party. I suppose I didn't realize how naïve I was or trusting of others. I just wanted to be like the other girls. They seemed to have something I didn't, but I wasn't quite sure what that was. Maybe they didn't have as many secrets as I did, or maybe their family life was different. They didn't always have houses as nice as ours, but they seemed more carefree.

Several of my friends smoked cigarettes. I thought it made them look older and cooler. My dad even started to smoke cigarettes around the house.

One day, Jeannette said she'd teach me how to smoke after school. *How does she know all this stuff?* I wondered. We met at our lockers, then walked down the alley about a half block from school before she pulled out cigarettes and matches. It was windy that day and after wasting almost a half of a pack of matches, we huddled between two garages to block the wind. Even when we stood close together, between the buildings, the matches kept going out, but eventually she lit her cigarette and then she used that cigarette to light another one. Just as she handed it to me, telling me to put it in my mouth and draw hard, a police car pulled up, and an officer jumped out of the car.

"Cop," I said. I dropped the cigarette and stepped on it.

"Shit." Jeannette dropped her cigarette and stomped on it as well.

"What are you two doing back here?" the officer inquired.

"Nothing," we said at the same time.

"The owner of the garage reported that you were lighting matches. He was afraid you were going to start a fire," he said in his best cop voice.

"We'd never do that," I said, my heart pumping fast in my chest.

"It smells like you've been smoking. What are your names and where do you live?" He pulled a notebook and a pencil from his breast pocket.

We took turns giving him our full name and address, visibly shaking.

"I will be calling your parents, so I suggest you go directly home."

"Okay," we mumbled and nodded, then while he watched, we headed home in opposite directions. Once his car passed me at the end of the alley, I ran the entire way home. I tried to catch my breath before I turned the front doorknob, prepared to get yelled at.

"Hi, how was school?" Mom asked cheerfully.

"Uh, good. It was good." I walked towards my bedroom. *The cop must not have called yet. Maybe when he does, I can pretend to be Mom. Then she'll never find out.* I hovered near the phone all night, but when ten o'clock rolled around, I realized he wasn't going to call. What a relief! The next day in school Jeannette told me no one had called her house either. The cop was just trying to scare us. And scare us he did. I forgot about smoking for a while.

That summer I bought a membership at the local swimming pool, but I went with my friends instead of my brother. I still swam daily after chores. Dad got a new job as a night shift security guard at the Coca-Cola plant they had just finished building in Hamburg. Mom still worked at Whitner's in the tearoom. She bought all my clothes there. I knew the clothes were expensive, but she explained it by saying the quality was much better and the clothes would last longer.

I started eighth grade, excited to reconnect with the friends I hadn't seen over the summer. Kevin was now in the high school in a different building. Mom usually took us to school in the morning and we both walked home. Math, Science, History, Art, and Home Economics were my favorite subjects. We typically didn't get a lot of homework, and if I used my study halls wisely, I could finish everything before the end of the school day. Mom knew how much I enjoyed sewing, so she bought me my first sewing machine, and I started to make all sorts of clothing for myself—skirts and tops. I already knew how to cook, but at school I learned some delicious deserts I made for my family.

Dad's heart problems continued. Mom was already cooking low-fat foods for all of us, but the doctors told Dad he needed to quit smoking and lose some weight. Because he ignored them for the most part, Mom and I both learned CPR through the American Heart Association, just in case.

Dad had had a sudden heart attack in the middle of the night that year. We were all at home in Shillington, sound asleep. Mom woke me up to help them until the ambulance arrived. We never had to use our CPR training, though we were ready to. Dad stayed alert and talking. He ended up in Coronary Care at the local hospital. From then on, Mom and Dad both decided he'd be better off going to the cardiologists at that hospital than those at the Veterans Administration. Mom thought the V.A. doctors had him taking too many drugs.

Another time in the summer of 1976 when I was still living at home in Shillington, Mom was working and Dad called for me down in my basement apartment. "Kim," he yelled. "Can you take me to the hospital?" The hospital was only about four miles from our house, so I suppose he figured that would be faster than waiting for an ambulance.

"The hospital? Why? Dad, what's wrong?"

He wouldn't say, but I assumed heart attack. Russ, the guy I was dating at the time, was also there. We got Dad into the back seat of my Ford Grand Torino

Once we got on the road, Dad said, "Put your flashers on and don't wait at traffic lights. If there's no traffic, just keep going." My dad was a man of few words, and that's all he said. That made me even more worried. Sure enough, when we got to the ER, he was admitted to coronary care for a heart attack.

All told, Dad had at least six heart attacks that began in his early forties before he agreed to open heart surgery in 1997 at age seventy-four, which turned out to be a quadruple bypass. He had never agreed to surgery because he was terrified of cardiac catheterization—threading a catheter through a vein in the arm, neck, or groin to examine the heart. He never said why, and I never understood. When I was a critical care nurse, cardiac catheterizations were done all day long just across the hall from our unit. By this time I had been married to Rod for more than fifteen years, and we were living with our children in Connecticut.

I went back to Pennsylvania by myself to help out. The surgery was a great success, so much so that he wished he had agreed to it earlier.

The fall was a mix of football games and sleepover parties at my girlfriends' houses. I had fun whenever I was out of the house. Boys were starting to like me, and my friends passed me notes in study hall or between classes to fill me in on the details. Some of the boys asked for my phone number, but I NEVER wanted a boy to call me at home. I didn't give my number out.

I felt as if I was finally fitting in. I stopped hanging out with Jeannette, instead spending time with a larger group of girls a year older than me. I had finally learned how to smoke as well, though I didn't inhale until I realized the gang made fun of another girl who didn't inhale, so I learned quickly. To me, it was all about fitting in.

One night Dad went to work but didn't come home. He had been doing his night rounds outside the Coca-Cola plant, unaware that a construction crew had dug a very deep hole and left it unbarricaded. The perimeter of the building was poorly lit, and the batteries in the flashlights had gone dead at the same time. He fell into the hole and hurt himself so bad, he spent the night there. The next morning, Dad caught the attention of the morning shift by throwing rocks out of the hole. By then, he was in shock. They called an ambulance and at the hospital, he immediately went into surgery with a compound fracture of his right leg. He stayed in the hospital for almost a week. When he came home, he was in a cast from his toes to his knee.

After a couple of days, Dad asked me to get him a clothes hanger. His leg itched, he explained. I watched as he carefully untwisted the metal hanger and stuck it down the length of his cast, moving it back and forth, homing in on the itch. I cringed, imagining what he must have been doing to his skin. This went on for several days, until we all noticed a putrid smell when we entered the room. We threw away the hanger and took him back to his surgeon. The leg had become badly infected, a real setback for him.

Dad had many problems with his leg over the next two and a half years. The fracture became non-union, which meant it wasn't joining together to heal. He required more surgery and pins to hold the bones together—and more casts. He became a recliner chair invalid, barking out orders like the Chief Warrant Officer he had recently been. He ran us all ragged. I felt like Cinderella without the glass slipper. As soon as I'd sit down, he'd ask for something else—a glass of water, more ice for his drink, a fluffier pillow, a less fluffy pillow. It wasn't just me. He did this to all of us, despite the fact that he had been fitted with a walking cast and had been instructed to walk as much as possible. It didn't matter. He didn't listen to anybody, and did whatever he wanted. While drinking one day (well, he drank just about every day), he noticed his toes were swelling. Instead of telling his doctor, he cut the cast off his leg himself. I didn't understand his logic, but I wasn't going to argue with my father, especially when he was drinking. I didn't know how Mom put up with him.

Once Dr. Morrow—Dad's surgeon and friend from high school—determined the bone still hadn't healed together, he performed bone grafting surgery on Dad's leg, put a new cast on him, and told him in no uncertain terms not to touch the cast again. I think Dad even listened to him that time!

CHAPTER 6

INNOCENCE LOST

In the spring of eighth grade, something happened to me that changed the course of my life, and not in a good way.

It began innocently enough.

It was just after lunch and like the rest of my class, I was heading to art. I was creative and art was one of my favorite subjects, even though I excelled in math and science as well.

I saw Brent walking towards me. He was a ninth grader, but whenever he passed me in the hall, he stared at me and tried to get my attention so he could say "Hi." He wasn't that cute. In fact, I didn't find him attractive at all. He was a teenaged boy, pimply and awkward, big without looking particularly athletic or muscular. But his attention intrigued me. Why would a ninth grader be interested in me, an eighth grader? Besides, I was new to this boy-girl thing and found myself unusually shy around boys. I wanted people to like me, so I usually went along with whatever they said.

Something was different that day, as if he wanted to do more than say hello. He motioned me to step aside. My heart pounded so hard I could feel it in my throat. My face grew hot as I turned red.

I said, "Hi," then tried to move past him, but he blocked my way. I looked at him as if to say, Okay, what is it?

He came right out with it. "Do you think you could go with me tonight to V & S to get a sandwich?"

This came out of the blue and took me by surprise. V & S was a sandwich store we all went to from time to time, but I had never gone with a boy before. My first thought was that Mom would never let me go out with this boy I barely knew and she didn't know at all. *How can I say no without looking like a fool?* Without thinking, I blurted, "Yes."

"Great," he said. "My friend Denny and I will pick you up at five-thirty."

I turned and headed to class without responding. I couldn't focus on very much else the rest of the day. All I could think was, *How am I going to get out of this? Why did I say, yes? My parents will never let me go, then everyone will laugh at me!*

As soon as school was over, I rushed home. I was on a mission. I took Mom aside, and I explained how Brent had asked me out. We both knew Denny. He lived a few blocks away, and Mom knew Denny's parents, so she assumed Denny was a nice young man, as she put it. She did not know Brent, though, and she asked me a lot of questions about him. I couldn't answer most of them. She said Dad would never let me to go in a car alone with two boys, even if it was just to get sandwiches and come directly home.

I wasn't giving up, so I asked her to ask Dad on my behalf while I waited in my room. I could hear their voices as they talked but couldn't make out any of it until I heard a very loud, "NO." How was I ever going to save face at school?

I was brave in my desperation, so I walked into the kitchen and said, "Please Dad, can I go? I'll come home as soon as we eat our sandwich." Then Mom reminded Dad that she knew Denny's parents and they were very nice people. "Please, please Dad. Let me go just this one time!"

He looked directly into my eyes, drawing out the silence that had descended on us in anticipation. Then he said, "Okay, you can go, but just this one time!"

I instantly felt relief. I wouldn't have to call Brent to say I couldn't go and look like a fool to a ninth grader. Since I had no real interest in Brent, after that night I'd explain that we were just friends, and then I'd make sure I'd NEVER find myself in this situation again. Now that it was going to happen, though, I got nervous all over again. *What would we talk about?* I really was very shy around boys, and whenever I got too nervous, I'd get blotchy red hives on my arms. *Oh, great. Something else to worry about.*

Mom called my name, maybe for the second or third time, and when she got my attention, she asked, "How much money do you need?"

We decided that five dollars would be plenty for a small sandwich and a soda. As I tucked the money into my pants pocket, the doorbell rang. I ran towards the door and in a loud voice said, "I'll get it!"

I opened the door, said, "Hi." I turned and yelled, "I'll be back soon." Then quickly shut the door before my parents could ask for introductions.

I walked to the light blue two-door Comet, Brent ahead of me. When he reached the car, he opened the front door and moved the front seat forward so I could get into the back seat. I acknowledged Denny by saying, "Hi." The windows were down because of the heat. As we pulled away, the breeze blew through my long hair, which I gathered in one hand to keep out of my face.

We turned the corner onto Sterley Street, and after a complete stop at the stop sign, Denny turned left. *Why did he turn left? He should have gone straight.* I was puzzling this out while trying to focus on the conversation. At the next stop sign, Denny turned right onto Wyomissing Boulevard. *Yep, that's the right way*, I told myself. But then the car slowed down and Denny turned left just before Wixon's Bakery onto a dirt road, and stopped. *Why did we stop here? This was not the plan! What's going on?* I was getting worried. How much could I trust these boys?

I almost didn't hear Brent when he turned and said, "Do you mind if we get out for a minute? I'd like to talk to you before we go to V & S."

Worry shifted to fear, and I couldn't answer. I thought about the promise I made to my parents, and this wasn't it. I was letting them down. Brent had already gotten out of the car and had pulled the seat forward for me, but something was telling me not to get out. I froze in place. Denny had turned to look at me, too. I felt uncomfortable under their gaze. I pushed the seat forward and squeezed through the small space.

Once out of the car, I followed Brent's lead, unsure of where we were going and why. About a hundred feet ahead the dirt road turned slightly to the right and from there you could see the abandoned concrete bridge, the stream moving rapidly beneath it. He reached out and took my hand. *Oh no*, I thought. *That's what this is about? I don't really like you.* I pulled my hand away, trembling. My heart pounded faster. The stream was right there, but the sound of the water seemed far away. The chirping of the birds receded as well. I was entering a kind of twilight zone. I walked more slowly, taking in my surroundings, looking for a way out. The only way out was back to Denny's car.

When we reached the edge of the bridge, he stopped and said, "Let's sit down for a minute. I'd like to talk with you."

I had on brand new yellow pants, and all I could imagine was how dirty they'd get if I sat on that old bridge. I looked at him, willing him to understand. Instead, he grabbed my hand and squeezed until it hurt, then pulled me down to sit next to him. I tried to pull away, but he held on tight. I was truly scared now.

As soon as I sat down, he leaned in and forced a kiss on me. I tried to lean away, but he pressed harder and harder against me. Stop, I wanted to yell, but I couldn't free my mouth. He was stronger than he looked and he had taken me by surprise. I felt weak against his advances. I wanted to stop it, but I couldn't. At least I felt like I couldn't. It was as if it was all happening to someone else.

My thoughts were a jumble: Why had my parents given in so easily? I thought about the promise I made to them, how my new clothing was going to be ruined, the cold bridge on which I was now lying on back. *When did I lie down? Where's Denny? Why isn't he helping me? Oh God, is he watching?*

Brent was on top of me now, his unexpected weight hurting me. I wanted to cry, but I was trying to be a big girl. He got hold of my zipper, pulled it down, then he pulled down my pants and my underwear. *What, why is he doing this?* I felt the bridge's rough concrete against my butt. He did something with his pants, then I felt an intense pain as if I was being stabbed down there. I couldn't put a name to what was happening, but I knew it was bad, really bad. I whimpered, crying silently to myself, but that only seemed to encourage him. *God, please make him stop. This hurts. This hurts. This hurts.* I try to think about anything but what was happening. I thought about my brother and parents at home, my happy place until recently. It really wasn't so bad after all. I thought about the painting I was working on in art class. Was that only this morning? I thought about the fun we used to have at my grandparents' farm. I thought about how I wished this could all be a nightmare that I'd soon wake up from. I thought about how I had always wanted to be a mother and how now I wasn't sure I'd be able to have children. Although I couldn't really articulate it just then, I somehow knew that everything had changed irrevocably. That my place in the world had changed.

Then suddenly he lifted himself off me and I was finally able to move. "Get dressed. We have to go," was all he said.

I was numb. I couldn't talk. I couldn't think. I followed his simple instructions.

We returned to the car in silence. I don't know how we got to V & S or what we talked about, if anything, on the ride. We walked into the sandwich shop, pausing just inside the door to take a number. I didn't want anyone to see my eyes, so I looked down. That's when I saw the patch of blood soaking through the crotch of my yellow pants.

Can everyone see this? Was it on the seat of my pants as well? My face turned red. I was certain that everyone in the shop could see exactly what had happened all over me, though I still wasn't quite sure myself what actually had happened. I turned my legs to hide the stain, but saw that would do nothing. My number was called. To my surprise, I stepped up to the counter, and ordered a small Italian sandwich on a hard roll, no onions, and a root beer without breaking into hysterical sobs.

I waited for my order, motionless, empty, sad, and confused. It seemed to take an extremely long time for the sandwich to be made and the fountain drink poured and both to be placed on the countertop. I slapped my five-dollar bill down on the counter, and reached for my change. I was sure that everyone was watching me as I walked briskly to the seat just in front of the window overlooking Lancaster Avenue and dropped into it. *Safe at last*, I thought. *At least for now.* By then Brent and Denny had joined me. Had they noticed the blood? Brent sat next to me, and Denny sat on the other side of Brent. They unwrapped their sandwiches and started to eat. How could they? I felt such revulsion I wanted to vomit.

"Aren't you hungry?" Brent asked.

"Not really, but I'll try," I said. I unwrapped my sandwich. I had to act as if nothing had happened, as if everything was normal. I had to force myself to eat so I could get home before my parents got suspicious. Tears welled in my eyes. I tried hard not to cry, but I did not succeed. I turned away from them—could I still call them boys?—so they wouldn't see the tears rolling down my cheeks. *Stop crying*, I told myself. *No one will ever know. Bite, chew, swallow. Bite, chew, swallow. Drink, swallow.* I tasted nothing. I enjoyed nothing. *Stop crying*, I scolded myself. *Stop crying right now!*

And with that, it was over. I wiped away the tears. I tucked away the pain, hate, and fear then and there. *Finish eating*, I said to myself. *Smile like nothing's wrong. Walk out behind the guys so they can't see your pants.*

I didn't talk on the drive home. All I could think about was how was I going to get into the house unnoticed to change clothes. The closer we got to the house, the more nervous I felt. Maybe eating that sandwich hadn't been a good idea. I was going to throw it up any second now. When the car stopped in front of the house, Brent stepped out and moved the seat forward. I pushed the seat hard, and moved through the opening like a wild animal freed from its cage.

But I wouldn't be free for a long time.

I barreled through the front door, and no one was in sight. I ran into my bedroom and stripped down. I grabbed clean underwear and jeans and got dressed again. I buried the soiled underwear and pants in the back of my closet under a pile of shoes and purses. My secret was safe for now.

I went into the bathroom and locked the door behind me, even though we never locked doors in our house. If Mom caught me with the door locked, she'd know something was wrong, but I didn't want anyone to barge in while I was cleaning up the blood.

I cleaned up without anyone noticing, then left the bathroom, and made it back to my room. I heard Mom's footsteps coming my way.

She poked her head through the door and said, "How was dinner?"

I wanted to cry and fall into her familiar embrace so she could make it all go away. But I knew I could never tell her—or anyone. I couldn't bring shame on the family. It would be a secret, my secret, forever. *Unless Brent or Denny opened their big mouths!* I realized with a jolt of fear. *They wouldn't, would they? What could I do about that?*

I couldn't look Mom in the eyes, but I pulled it together enough to get out, "It was fine. I just ate and came home."

"Do you have homework tonight?" she asked.

"Nope. Finished it in study hall." Mom seemed satisfied with that. I slowly closed my door, and heard her walk away. *A plan*, I thought. *I need a plan!*

The underwear was easy. When I was sure Mom and Dad were watching TV in the living room, I made my way toward the kitchen.

Kevin was doing his homework at the dining room table. I was in the clear. I didn't waste a second and quietly stuffed the underwear deep into the trash, rearranging some paper on top to make sure it was well hidden.

But what about the pants? I only wore them once! Mom always did the laundry, and I didn't know how to use the washer or how to get stains out of clothes. I thought about it for a bit. Maybe I could dye the pants! That might work! A dark color would hide the blood and I could just say I didn't like yellow pants! Dye couldn't cost that much, could it? Back in my room, I fished some bills and change out my piggy bank to take with me the next day.

I got into bed, but couldn't sleep. After a while everyone was sleeping except me. The house grew dark, silent, and still. Questions came at me like a jackhammer. *What could I have done—should I have done—to stop it? Did I dress the wrong way? Why did I say yes? I really didn't want to go! Why did I trust someone I didn't know? Why didn't Denny help me? Was he in on it? Will my parents find out? Are kids at school going to treat me differently? Would I ever be able to forget? Am I ever going to be able to have children?* A million more questions raced through my mind with no answers until I fell asleep from exhaustion.

As always, Mom woke me up with a hearty "Good morning!" I was jittery, guilt-ridden, and filled with impending doom.

I hoped I wouldn't see Brent in school. I never wanted to see him again, but I didn't know how to avoid him, and sure enough, after lunch, he came up behind me without warning and whispered, "You should have told me you were a virgin." I nearly jumped out of my skin. The only sex education I ever had was of the your-bodies-are-changing-and-you'll-need-to-use-deodorant variety, so I had no clue what he was talking about. I didn't say anything, then disappeared into the safety of my next class.

After school, I picked up some fabric dye from the pharmacy, Burnt Umber, and walked home fast. I figured I had just over an hour. Dad was watching TV from his usual chair, while I retrieved the bloody pants and took them to the basement laundry room. I read the instructions, then found our red bucket, which I filled halfway with hot water. Knowing that this would be the last time I'd see the blood, I submerged the pants in the water with relief. I could breathe again!

I waited for twenty minutes, poking at the pants with a mop handle to make sure the dye was even. I left them in a few minutes longer than required just in case, then wrung the water from the pants as I snaked them out of the bucket. The pants were now the color of dried blood! So much for trying to forget. Here was a sick and sickening reminder, my very own scarlet letter.

I hung the pants on a hanger in my closet until they were good and dry, then took them to Mom to show her what I had done. She was bound to see them anyway.

"Oh my God, Kim, what did you do to your new pants? You've ruined them!" Mom said.

I lied that I didn't care for yellow pants once I wore them, so I dyed them a different color. The truth was, the pants were ruined—shrunken and blotchy—and I was never going to wear them again. I couldn't stand the sight of them. I also couldn't throw them out after my elaborate lie, so I folded them neatly and placed them in a corner on my closet floor, where they remained out of sight for years until Mom cleaned out our closets and added them to the donation pile.

As much as I prayed for that to be the end, my ordeal wasn't over—not even close. Brent took over my life. Literally. He didn't even pretend we were boyfriend and girlfriend. I was his—I don't know what to call it without being crude. Let's just say I was at his disposal. He owned me.

At first, it just seemed like a series of coincidences. I'd be out with friends and he'd show up, and he'd take me off somewhere, and—let's call it what it was—rape me. I couldn't say no. I was afraid to say no. After this happened a couple of times, I wondered how he knew where I was all the time. Was there a spy? Were my friends telling him our plans, or did he find out on his own? I never knew. But he was always there. I lived in constant fear of the next time he'd find me. Why didn't I just stay home? That was not an option. I was a teenager, after all, longing desperately to fit in, and home had its own problems, with Dad's drinking and erratic behavior.

I kept going out. He kept finding me. He kept raping me, time and time again.

I was a thirteen-year-old girl, afraid and confused. Afraid doesn't even cover it. I was *terrified*. I had descended into my own personal hell. Nothing mattered anymore. As I saw it, my life was over. I prayed that God would tell Mom what was going on or that she'd find out some other way so she could stop it somehow. All I knew was that I couldn't tell her—I couldn't bear the thought of the immense pain that would bring her.

I hung out with older kids. Some form of alcohol was almost always available—beer, wine, sometimes the harder stuff and some-times weed—but until Brent, I could take it or leave it. After Brent—it was my lifeline. It was the old cliché, I drank to forget, to numb myself to the terror and the pain. From the first sip, I drank like an alcoholic. I didn't stop until I blacked out, and when I blacked out, I couldn't remember what happened. That was how I got through those nights with Brent.

One night when I knew Brent would find me, I drank a fifth of whiskey. It did the job. I was stumbling, blackout drunk, and I don't remember much of that night. Mom filled me in on some of it, and the rest I figured out. What I do remember is that at some point after being sexually violated, someone—I have no idea who—drove me home, propped me against the front door, rang the doorbell, then sped off.

Mom always waited up for me. When she answered the door, I fell into the house. "Shh, don't wake your father," she whispered, trying to pull my dead weight to my feet. She didn't have to worry about Dad. The cardiac protocol had him on heavy sedation, and despite all the noise I made that night, Dad slept on peacefully.

When Mom finally got me upright, I pinballed down the hallway until, fully dressed, I passed out face down on my twin bed. Throughout the night, I woke only long enough to vomit into my hair and pillow. Mom came in and cleaned me up each time.

This next part is embarrassing, but I've vowed to tell it all. At some point during the night, I had to use the bathroom—to evacuate my bowels, as we say in the nursing profession. I got out of bed, but I was still drunk and not thinking clearly. Disoriented and on my knees, I crawled through the first door I saw—my closet, it turns out. I took my father's reel-to-reel tape recorder for a toilet, and you can imagine the rest. Then I somehow got back into bed.

I woke up the next afternoon with the worst pounding headache of my life. I closed my eyes against the sunlight and sobbed in pain. Mom stepped into the room telling me how sick I had been, but after only a few words, I vomited again, this time into the bucket she had placed next to my bed. I vomited throughout the rest of that day into the evening, which made the headache worse. I couldn't open my eyes. Mom offered me fluids, but the thought only made me vomit more violently. Mom told Dad I had the flu, which he seemed to believe, though the room must have reeked of booze.

The room also reeked of a disgusting odor I couldn't identify, an odor that made me vomit even more. By late afternoon I couldn't take it any longer, and I begged Mom to figure out what it was. It took a while, but once she opened the closet door, it was clear what the problem was. She took the recorder into the basement, then cleaned up the closet floor and just about hosed down the room with air freshener. The chemical smell made me gag a little too, but it was immensely better than the alternative.

Mom came through for me that weekend, but when she finished cleaning up, she had this to say: "When you feel better, you have to clean the recorder. That'll be your punishment for doing something so stupid."

And that's exactly what I did several days later. I will never forget how disgusting it was to clean up the recorder, with the poop dried by then and stuck in all the little crevices. *If only I could tell her why I had drunk so much*, I thought, the whole time I was cleaning the device. But in our family, you didn't talk—you kept secrets. Grandma kept recipe secrets, Mom kept childhood secrets, Dad kept war secrets. We all had our own secrets, and I guessed I now had mine too.

I never drank whiskey again, but I didn't stop drinking, and I didn't stop drinking to black out, beer and wine mostly. It was the only way I could get through it. The hard rock music of the day was the soundtrack to most of the parties where Brent found me—Jimi Hendrix, Led Zeppelin, Grand Funk Railroad. I came to hate that music for what it reminded me of, and I threw all my albums into the trash so I'd feel safe in my own home.

One day he found me before I had a chance to drink. I don't remember where it was, maybe an ice cream parlor or something like that. I wanted to run, but there was no place to go he wouldn't follow me. Frightened and afraid, virtually unable to breathe, I started praying, and whether it was the rhythm of the words or the fact that my mind had turned inward, I left my body and drifted away. I was physically present without being mentally present. I pictured happier times and places—playing on my Grandparents' farm, the cool water of a good summer swim, learning something new and exciting at school. Having done some research now as an adult, I know that most people undergoing something traumatic do this in some form or other—it's called dissociation—but to me it was a miracle, one that worked almost as well as alcohol.

Why didn't I just tell him no? It's difficult to say precisely what I was thinking as a thirteen-year-old, but looking back, I think it was shame and fear. Shame that I was letting him do these things to me, even though I didn't feel as if I had a choice, and fear of what he would do to me and our family if I said no. He told me that if I ever tried to get away from him, he would hurt me bad, and everyone I cared about.

And I believed him. He was bigger and stronger than me, and cruel, lacking something essential that would have made him human.

He took control of me in other ways. One night he took me to his house, which terrified me until I realized his parents were home. *What could happen with his parents home?* I thought. I grew afraid again when he told them we were going into his room and they said, "Okay."

Once upstairs, he shut the door behind us and showed me a pair of knee-high suede boots with fringes on the back. "Try them on," he commanded.

I tried them on, as he knew I would, and a shiver of fear went through me. They fit perfectly. How did he know my size? This was a new level of creepy. He reminded me of what he would do to me and my family if I resisted him, then forced me to have sex with him—raped me—with more enthusiasm than usual. Apparently the boots did something for him.

My heart raced. My stomach churned. The sight of his pimples, tipped and shiny with puss, made me gag. *Swallow, swallow*, I told myself. Who knew what he would do if I threw up just then. I took a deep breath to calm my stomach, closed my eyes, and floated away on big, white fluffy clouds towards the rainbow in the distance. *Ah, that's better. You're not there, you're here, drifting toward happy.*

"Hey," he said, shaking my shoulder. "You can go now."

When he was done, he was done, and it was over. *Safe for now! Safe for now!* I repeated to myself. *Safe for now!* I pulled up my jeans and straightened my top, sat on the bed to take off the boots I was still wearing.

"Leave them on," he ordered. "And wear them to school. Every day."

I didn't even argue, I was so eager to get out of that house.

Other weird things were happening. Out of nowhere one day, I heard a chorus of hundreds of people screaming in my head. I couldn't make out actual words, just shrieks and stormy confusion. It didn't happen every day, but it continued sporadically after that first time. The cacophony lasted about a minute, and it always scared me, the sound of demons in a horror movie. But this was no movie, and the demons were my own.

I didn't tell anyone about the voices at first, but they went on for months, and it was driving me crazy. I finally told Mom. She thought about it, looking concerned. Then she said she wasn't sure why this was happening to me, but the next time it did, I should pray to God to take it away.

I followed Mom's advice, and it worked! One day I realized the voices had stopped, and they never visited me again.

But Mom had no solution for another problem I was having. As much as I had enjoyed school when I was younger, it meant nothing to me anymore. In fact, I hated it. I hated it because that's where I met him, and I had to see him every day. It became a prison. I woke up every morning sick to my stomach with fear. Some days I pretended I really was sick just so I didn't have to go to school.

My grades plummeted, but no one noticed until I got my first D.

Mom spoke with me privately. "You seem more interested in boys than schoolwork," she said. "That's not like you."

She must have known about Brent. Did she seriously think I liked him? Others had said much the same, wondering if we were boyfriend and girlfriend. That made me want to puke. I didn't know much, but I knew we weren't that. We didn't hold hands at the movies, we didn't go skating, we didn't watch TV on the couch. What we did was a lot less—innocent. I wanted to cry out, *HELP ME, MOM. DON'T YOU SEE WHAT'S REALLY GOING ON?* I so wanted to tell her. I so wanted not to have to tell her, that she would somehow just magically know what was going on and swoop in and save me and make it all better. I guess that's why it's called magical thinking.

Instead, I said, "I really don't think that's the problem. School's just getting harder."

"Maybe you should study more," she said.

"Yep, I will," I said, before retreating to the safety of my bedroom.

I quietly closed and locked the door behind me, then sobbed and sobbed. If it was only that simple. If only I could tell her, then I might be free, the nightmare would be over. But it was too late for that. I could never tell her. It would break her, or so I thought. I'm a people pleaser, I always want people to be happy. Except me. I didn't deserve to be happy. I climbed into bed, said my prayers, and cried myself to sleep.

CHAPTER 7

SAVED BY THE NEW KID IN TOWN

One thing I could be happy about was that school ended for the year and Brent would be moving on to the high school. We wouldn't be in the same school anymore!

But that didn't change things as much as I hoped it would. He still showed up at many of the places and parties I went to, and took me off into a room or hiding place and raped me. I hated it, but I felt helpless to stop it. Anyone else who has been through this understands why. Remember, he had threatened to hurt me and my family and I believed him.

I felt helpless to stop it until I met the person who gave me the strength I needed to stand up for myself, not by anything she said but simply by who she was.

As I did every summer, I joined the public swimming pool. I planned to meet friends at the pool on one of the first swim days, but I was so eager, I arrived long before they did and saved my spot on the ground with a beach towel that covered my purse. I had brought along a new tube of Prell, and I didn't want anyone to make off with it. When we were in the military, Dad didn't make enough money for us to buy shampoo. We washed our hair with Dove soap. Now I got an allowance and could purchase my own shampoo and conditioner.

While waiting at the entrance for my friends, I noticed a self-confident girl about our age get dropped off out front. I heard her mom holler, "Have fun and make some friends," just before she closed the door.

She must be new, I thought. She had that "it" quality about her, and I wanted to get to know her. Once she paid and came through the enterance, I introduced myself.

She told me her name was Shelley, and she had just moved from Syracuse, New York. She was the same age as I was and going into ninth grade in the fall. I asked her to sit with me, so I could introduce her to some of my friends. After a short while, we realized we had much in common. We were both raised in middle class homes, and our parents had similar values. Her dad, Johnny, had served in WWII and her brother, Jack, had served in Vietnam. Her mom and Terry were both nurses. We both smoked cigarettes and pot and drank. Because we seemed older than our classmates, we both dated older guys.

After talking for a while, I asked her if she had any plans for the evening, and when she didn't, I said, "Why don't we hang out together?" That evening, I met her parents and she met mine. Shelley was unlike any friend I had ever had before. She was outgoing and smart, not afraid to stand up for herself. She didn't play games. I envied that about her, wanted to be more like her.

We became instant best friends. Once I met Shelley, I let some of my previous friendships fall away (the toxic ones, we would say today, the ones that enabled Brent's behavior), and made friends with a group of new, more genuine people who came into Shelley's orbit.

I didn't tell Shelley anything about Brent, but I started to look at how I imagined Shelley might see him. She wouldn't have put up with him, I was sure, and seeing it this way gave me the confidence to hope for something different, to imagine a life without him in it.

SAVED BY THE NEW KID IN TOWN | **85**

If I had just half the strength Shelley had, I could do it. With Shelley as my role model and source of empowerment, I dug deep and found the strength to confront Brent a few days after he had raped me one night that summer—for the last time.

I was beyond petrified when I picked up the phone and stretched the long cord onto the cellar steps before dialing his number. His little sister answered, and he picked up a few seconds later. Before I could chicken out, I spoke quickly but with conviction. I was no longer the naive virgin he had conquered! I let him know that we were through; that I didn't want to see him or hear him or even hear about him again; that if ever came near me again, I would tell everyone what he had done to me, starting with the police. I don't remember if he even said anything to defend himself because I didn't leave much time between sentences.

When I finished, I slammed the receiver with such force I thought I had broken it. I was glad no one was home. My whole body was shaking with the rush of adrenalin. I smiled at my next idea. I walked into my bedroom, opened the closet, and gathered up those awful boots, the symbol of his perverse control of me. I marched out the side door, lifted the trashcan lid, and stuffed those ugly boots as deep in the garbage as I had my bloodied underwear the day this had all got started. I laughed out loud. *I am free at last. I will never let anything like this happen again.* I took a deep breath, and as I blew it out, I felt as if I had been reborn.

It had taken six long months to get to this point, but thanks to Shelley, I did it. I wish I could have told her what she had done for me, but I was too embarrassed to share my deepest, darkest secret, even with my new best friend.

And that was that. My threat to go to the police was enough to keep him away. I wished I had done it sooner. Once I was in high school, I ignored him whenever I saw him, though his presence in the same building was a constant reminder of what had happened and was a big factor in my feelings of shame and worthlessness throughout high school.

I did talk to Brent one more time. This was in 1978, three years after I graduated from high school. I was in Johnny's Cafe, standing at the bar to buy a round of drinks for my friends, and he came up on me from behind and said, "Hi Kim, do you remember me?"

I jumped. Flashback. In my head I screamed, *How the fuck could I EVER forget what you did to me?* Instead I played it cool, at least as cool as I could. "Yes, I do, and please leave me alone." I returned to my friends. If he would have tried anything, my guy friends would have had my back. They were all much bigger than him! At that point, he no longer scared me; he repulsed me.

+ + +

Shelley and I were inseparable that summer. In addition to the pool, a bunch of us swam at Monocacy, an abandoned quarry filled by underground springs of near freezing water. People jumped from the rocks along the sides into the deep water. We also went to nighttime outdoor parties with huge bonfires to keep us warm, and local concerts were held in a park nearby. When Shelley went back to Syracuse with her father, I went with them and met the friends she had been telling me about.

My parents loved Shelley, and Shelley's parents became second parents to me. Shelley's dad, Johnny, taught me some of his family's Russian Orthodox traditions, as well as some Russian phrases such as "I love you" and "Shut up." He loved how quickly I learned. The four parents became friends, and spent time at each other's homes for drinks, dinner, and cards.

Once school started, Shelley and I found out we didn't have classes together, but we didn't let that stop us. Every morning before school we walked to Yonner's Store for some penny candy, and sometimes we had lunch together at school. After school we walked to Rite Aid for a milk shake or an ice cream float at the soda counter. If we didn't go to Rite Aid, we went to Hardee's to hang out with other friends.

On the weekends, we went to a football or basketball game (depending on the season), and sometimes to a drinking party. Now when I drank, I didn't drink to oblivion; it was more social. I owed that to Shelley and our new group of friends. They helped me realize I no longer needed to accept anything but respect from the guys we now called friends.

We stayed busy that winter as well. We'd go sledding when it snowed, and when the local ponds froze, we'd go ice skating.

Though Shelley enjoyed our friendship, I found that she wasn't happy with Pennsylvania, and wanted to move back to Syracuse. It was late spring when Shelley told me her parents had decided to move back to Syracuse as soon as she finished school. I understood, sort of, but I was still heartbroken. How could she leave me and all her other new friends behind? She was my rock. She made me a better person. Would I ever find another friend like her?

The answer came more quickly than I thought it would. I had joined the track team that spring, and when we didn't have meets, we practiced every day. Even as a ninth grader, I was the second fastest sprinter on the team. If I had quit smoking, I probably would have been even faster, but I wasn't about to do that! I ran the fifty and the one hundred and was on the 440 relay team. We set records that season throughout the county.

That's how I met Gooker, who was also on the team. Her given name was Caroline, but no one called her that. The area of Pennsylvania we lived in had a large Pennsylvania Dutch contingent. In fact, my mother and her parents spoke Pennsylvania Dutch to each other when they didn't want us to understand what they were saying. "Gooker" in Dutch means "looker," at least that was my understanding. Her family called her Gooker because she was very inquisitive as a child, looking everywhere, and it stuck. Even though she was a year older than I was, we ran together at practice and afterwards, and she drove me home in Bessy, her car. Gooker was outgoing, funny, and easy to like. I met some of her other friends as well.

When ninth grade ended, it was time for Shelley and her parents to move back to Syracuse. Even though Shelley was excited to return, this was a sad time for me, and my parents hated to see their new friends leaving as well. We all spent one last evening together before they moved. Mom cooked, and they visited the entire night. No one wanted to be the first to say good-bye, but eventually, with lots of tears (at least for the girls), we finally parted.

Hurricane Agnes bore down on our county the day Shelley and her parents left. How fitting. Torrential rain pummeled the area and the local rivers swelled and overflowed their banks. When the rain finally stopped, my brother and his friends said they were going tubing on Wyomissing Creek. When Mom found out, she was furious. All she could imagine were headlines about drowned teenagers. She asked me to ride to the creek to stop them before they got in the water. I pedaled frantically to the Wyomissing Creek, all the while thinking it would be my first time back there since I was raped.

When I got there, I didn't find my brother and friends, but I saw something else that astonished me. The bridge was gone! The force of the rapids must have torn it away. I cried. The bridge was gone, the place I was raped, the symbol of all that had happened afterward. *Gone forever*, I whispered to myself. One day I hoped to be washed just as clean.

As the raging waters roared past, I saw beautiful purple wildflowers in bloom on the banks. I picked a handful and tossed them in the water, which snatched them away and took them downstream. My friend was gone and so was the bridge where I lost my innocence. I grieved for my friend and my innocence, then remounted my bicycle and rode home.

At home, my brother and his friends were sitting around the kitchen table, eating chips and cookies. They had decided not to brave the raging water after all. *Good choice*, I thought, wishing I could have done the same.

CHAPTER 8

HIGH SCHOOL GIRLS JUST WANT TO HAVE FUN

O nce high school started, I hung out with Gooker and her friends, who had a year of high school behind them. On weekends, we cruised Penn Street for hours, looping over to Franklin Street and back. It's what you did if you were a teenager and had a car or knew someone who did, a mobile party. We called out the windows to the other cars as we passed by.

Everyone thought I looked older than fifteen. For kicks one Friday night we tested the hypothesis by sending me into a bar in Reading to buy beer. Joy gave me her mom's fur coat to wear, and I added red lipstick. I'm sure we thought this was a brilliant idea for making me look older, but I probably just looked ridiculous, a child playing in her mother's clothes. They dropped me off at the bar, then circled the block. The room was dim and filled mostly with men. They all turned to look at me, and I almost bolted there and then, but I couldn't let my friends down. I casually smiled and walked up to the bartender.

"What can I get you?" he said, trying not to smirk.

"Two six packs of Pabst, please."

He raised an eyebrow, but turned to the large fridge and pulled out two six packs, one in each hand. *Thank God, he didn't ask for an ID. Stay calm. Stay calm.* He put the beer in a brown paper bag and told me what I owed him. I handed him a twenty. He put the change on the bar, and winked. I slid a dollar his way, smiled, said, "Thank you." I had fooled nobody, but I didn't care. He let me get away with it, and that's all that mattered.

When the car pulled up, I raised the bag to show them my prize, and they hooted and hollered. We'd have beer for the cruise! Once inside, I passed around a beer each to Gooker, Joy, and Maxine. "Let's get out of here," I said.

Back on Penn Street, a car full of older guys from Mifflin High School pulled up next to us when we stopped at a traffic light. Gooker grabbed a can from the bag and tossed it into their car. They yelled, "Throw us some more." But we just laughed as Gooker pulled away when the light changed. We had earned that beer!

We tried a different bar next time, this one in Angelica, along the Morgantown Road. It was dark when we pulled into the gravel lot on the side and out of view of the windows and front door. I put on the fur coat and lipstick. Inside I noticed this bar was less crowded than the other one, with only a few patrons seated on the barstools. I felt conspicuous, but I was committed. I walked to the bar and placed my order. Someone at the bar was buying a round of drinks for everyone. The bartender asked me what I wanted. I shrugged and said, "Pabst." I took a few sips and raised my glass to the man who bought the round.

As I enjoyed the cold draft, someone tapped me on the shoulder. I turned to see who it could be, expecting to see one of my friends. It was my Uncle Eugene, Mom's brother.

"Hello Kim," he said.

My heart skipped a few beats. "Uncle Eugene!" I whispered, then put my finger on my lips and said, "Shhhhh! Don't tell Mom."

"I won't," he said skeptically, asking with his eyes why in God's name I was doing this.

"Thanks," I said, taking my six packs from the bar. I was mortified I'd been caught, but I sure wasn't going to forget the beer.

As soon as I got into the car, I slapped the back of the seat and said, "Go. Go. Uncle Eugene saw me."

"What?" someone said.

"What happened?" someone else asked.

"Freaked me out. I asked him not to tell Mom, and he said he wouldn't." I opened the bag and passed a can to everyone. "Here's to Mom not finding out." I lifted my can in the air. "Cheers!"

As far as I know, my uncle never said a word. You can be sure we never went back to that bar, though.

Although I had reduced my drinking under Shelley's influence, Gooker and I just egged each other on, and this got us into more than a little trouble.

Before one Friday night football game, the cheerleading coach recruited Gooker to dress as the Mustang mascot to run onto the field at halftime and chase off the Muhlenberg Mule. She'd be the head, but she needed a partner to be the horse's behind. Of course, she thought of me, and I said, "Sure, why not? How hard can it be?"

She picked me up with a six-pack on the passenger seat. We found a place to stop on the way, and because we didn't have much time, we shotgunned three cans each. By the time we got to the stadium, we were very drunk and very silly, and could barely pay attention to the game.

Just before half time, we fumbled into our costume, and when they gave us the signal, we ran onto the field to chase the mule. Before we reached the middle of the field, however, the head dropped over Gooker's eyes and she couldn't see anything. I didn't know that, so when she stopped to fix it, I banged into her and knocked her over, then fell on top of her. We were still tipsy from the beer, and rolled on the ground giggling. Because we were stuck in the costume, we couldn't get up. We struggled on the ground for quite a while before we got to our feet. At that point, we said the heck with the mule and ran off the field to make way for the marching band.

Later, Gooker was fired from being the mascot.

"No shit?" we both said, then giggled some more.

My grades continued to drop. Instead of getting As and Bs, I was now a solid C student. I told myself that if I put more time into studying, I could get As any time I wanted to. But by then I didn't care. All I cared about was getting out of the house and partying with my friends. By junior year, Kevin was four hours away at college, and I didn't particularly like being the only kid in the house. I did have the entire basement apartment to myself, though. When I had friends over, we had as much privacy as we wanted, and Dad's dozen wine kegs were twenty feet away.

One morning I awoke to the most awful news. Some friends had been in a serious car accident. The Jeep they were driving in had unexpectedly flipped over, leaving Christopher severely injured. Maxine, Chris's girlfriend; another female passenger; and the driver, Doug, were all okay. They were treated and released from the hospital. Christopher however, required surgery to reduce the swelling in his brain. After surgery, he remained comatose on life support in intensive care.

We held a prayer vigil for Chris, but nothing we did seemed to help. He died soon after, and we were devastated, as if our whole world had ended. None of us were prepared for something like this. Dying was for old people. We were going to live forever. As his girlfriend, Maxine took it the hardest. We all tried our best to help her, but we were grieving as well.

How do you justify a young life snuffed out? Max and Chris had been dating for years and were planning on getting married someday. Now that would never happen, and a beautiful family had lost their son forever. There wasn't a dry eye at the funeral.

After the funeral, I had a heart-to-heart with God. *Heavenly Father, please bring Christopher into your presence today. Nurture and care for him, Lord. But could you also let me know he is safe with you in Heaven? You made today such a beautiful sunny day. Could you give us seven more beautiful Sundays in a row just like this one? Then on the eighth Sunday, let the weather change to allow me to see You and know that Chris is in your hands.*

I had never before made a request like this of the Lord, and never did again. This is not how the Lord works. Nor did I tell anyone else about my prayer. Meanwhile, I watched and waited.

The following Sunday was another beautiful beginning to the week, and so was every Sunday that followed, each one more beautiful than the last. The seventh Sunday was perhaps the most beautiful of all, with the softest of breezes and a spectacularly colorful light show of a sunset. Truly a sign from God!

I waited with my fingers crossed for the eighth Sunday.

As the weekend approached, the forecast changed. On Sunday it poured all day, with a hailstorm and the wind ripping branches from our small trees. I was never so happy to see a storm like this, one that showed the full might and glory of God. I knew then with all my being that Chris was with the Lord. The next time I saw Maxine, she talked about her wrenching loss and how she wasn't sure she could go on without Chris. I told her about my deal with God and how it had worked out, and she took some comfort in that.

It may seem a contradiction to some, but we prayed as hard as we partied, and my faith in God increased tremendously with the results of these prayers for Chris and the loved ones he left behind.

I had a part-time job at Spencer Gifts at the Berkshire Mall working with a girl named Val, who had already graduated from Wilson High, our rival, but that didn't get in the way of our friendship.

Our assistant manager was Mrs. Walters. "Tits" Walters, we called her when she wasn't around, a fifty-something transplant from the

1950s, with her overdone eyeliner, red lips, bleached blonde hair, chipped red nicotine-stained fingernails, and huge pointed bras. She chain-smoked nonfiltered Camels, and doused herself in dime store scent, a bad combination of smells that made us keep our distance when we could and breathe through our mouths when we couldn't. She treated us fairly well, and wasn't the worst boss in the world. I think she saw her younger self in us and lived vicariously through the adventure stories we told her in the slow times.

One night while working, a customer recommended trying Heister's in Reading, a bar and lounge that had live music and dancing every weekend. We both looked and acted older than we were, so we gave it a shot after work one Saturday night. We had so much fun we became regulars. Sometimes we'd go there directly after work, and other times we'd end up there after a night of club hopping. We'd drive there in Val's buttercup yellow Bug, blasting her Dolby Speakers with the Eagles or Boz Scaggs while singing along and smoking Val's dynamite weed.

John was the club's owner, and he took a liking to Val and me. I'm pretty sure he knew we were underage, but he didn't seem to care. We spent a good bit of money there, and it was rumored he was associated with the Mob, so nobody messed with him.

He never made us pay a cover unless his wife was working the door, and he always protected us from jerks and scumbags. He assigned his bodyguard and bouncer, Lou-Lou—the biggest, baddest-assed, Black man you'd ever want to meet—to look after us. Lou-Lou spoke slowly, almost shyly in a deep voice, but you didn't want to cross him. Lou-Lou even went with us to the after-hours bars after Heister's closed up for the night.

We also became friends with the bartenders, Bobby and Ray. Bobby usually had a supply of drugs and offered us coke or crank or pot, among others. Sometimes we accepted, sometimes we declined, though we soon figured out that when we snorted Bobby's drugs, we could drink much more than normal. Either way, we danced the night away. The bump was the most popular, perhaps because it was the easiest, consisting of the partners literally bumping their hips together suggestively. We wore the shortest of skirts or shorts and the tightest of bellbottoms to enhance our—bumping.

We did mostly recreational drugs, but we were open to just about anything. One weekend we joined Maxine to attend an overnight party in Boston. We got there early, and to give us something to do, Max's friend gave us magic mushrooms—psilocybin. We were a little nervous at first, but eventually we all tried some. What I remember most was lying for hours on a grassy green hill staring at cloud formations until I saw Abraham Lincoln's face. When I pointed him out, everyone else saw him too, and we laughed and laughed. We were late for the party we lay there so long, but to us, it was as if only minutes had passed.

In the summer on the weekends, my friends and I would get up a carful of girls and go to Wildwood, a legendary South Jersey shore town on a barrier island with a two-mile boardwalk and pristine beaches that went on forever. We'd go to the beach each day by nine, and stay until we turned four shades darker or were close to fainting with hunger. Then we'd go back to the motel, clean up, eat at one of the seafood shacks, and, since we all had fake IDs, hit the clubs at night.

It seemed an idyllic, carefree existence, but Val's life wasn't all sunshine and roses. Val had it rough at home—her father beat her, and her mother did nothing to stop it. Her mother was as afraid of the six-four father as Val was.

Val was an only child. Her father, John, wanted more children, but her mother did not. John was a gifted metallurgist who ran the metallurgy department at a specialty steel company. He was an exacting scientist and expected perfection from his only child. Unfortunately, Val had a learning disability and didn't understand math. She didn't pass a single math class in her time in school, even with the accommodations for her disability. Her father couldn't accept that she couldn't learn math. It didn't make him sad and disappointed—it made him angry, and he took it out on her, trying to control her every breath and beating her whenever she got out of line, as he saw it.

She told me about a night she walked past him while he was sitting in his recliner. She was listening to her cassette player. Her father said, "I'd like to use that sometime."

Val, being a smart-ass teenager, said, "Then get your own."

Her father jumped out of the recliner and chased her up the five steps to her bedroom. She made it to her room and locked the door, but her dad was a large man and broke the door down in a second. She stood in the middle of her room. He ran to her and punched her in the face. She lost her balance and fell to floor. He got on top of her and punched her again and again. When he wore himself out, he grabbed a handful of her long blonde hair and dragged her across the room until a hunk of hair came off in his hand. She had bald patches for months after that.

After nights like these, Val would show up at work or our house scabbed and bruised. Our hearts went out to her knowing there was nothing we could do. Ours wasn't the only family with dark secrets. Maybe that's why we were drawn to each other.

For my sixteenth birthday, Mom and Dad gave me a dark blue Ford Grand Torino and since my friends (other than Val) didn't have cars, I drove everywhere. As a senior, I hung out with Katie, Eileen, and Peggy at school, and Val joined us at night and on the weekends.

I picked up my school friends in the morning and took them home after school. Katie always had the best weed, which we smoked on the way to school, and sometimes finished in the parking lot. We thought we were so cool. Mom knew I smoked cigarettes, drank beer, and went to bars, but she had no clue I smoked pot, and I tried to keep it that way.

Katie and I joined a group of students who went to elementary schools at lunchtime to tutor the younger children. On our first day, we went to lunch at McDonald's instead of going to the assigned school. When no one back at our school seemed to notice, we made this a habit. Once a week we'd try a new place for lunch. We signed out in the principal's office when we left, and we signed in when we returned, just as we did when we actually went to the schools. The principal, who never caught on, always thanked us for our service. Well, we did provide service four out of five days.

On some of the days we played hooky, we went to Friendly Ice Cream, and other days we just drove around town, smoking pot. The afternoons were always easier to get through stoned. I hated school by then and all it stood for, I told myself—rules, authority, convention, achievement. What did it all matter? I know now that I was crying for help, so damaged and shamed by the trauma I endured that I just wanted to be numb. I thought this was how I could take back some control.

For spring break 1975, my parents splurged so I could go on our Senior Class Trip to Germany, Switzerland, and Austria. My only other close friend to go was Peggy, and we arranged to room together in advance.

Our first stop was Rothenberg, Germany, where we were dropped off by our double-decker tour bus. On the street I made a quick left turn and bumped into Dave Adams, literally. He was a U.S. soldier with some leave time, just a little older than we were, and lived on the outskirts of town. My friends and I invited him for a few beers, and he eagerly agreed. Because of the local customs—there was no real drinking age in Germany—alcohol was even easier to come by there. In fact, most of our parents signed a waiver permitting us to drink on the trip.

A few beers became many, and Dave missed the last train out. Since he had nowhere else to stay, we hid him in one of the boy's rooms. The four chaperones must have suspected something was going on, because at the last minute, they did a surprise room check and head count. But we had years of experience fooling teachers and parents, and were always a step or two ahead. We distracted the inspectors with some question or other, and moved Dave from room to room until the search was over. After lights out, Dave Adams, another Dave, and Mike knocked on our door, and we let them in. We laughed about our stupid teachers and how easy it had been to fool them. Mike was in his tighty whiteys, and mock posed for our camera before sneaking back to his room.

Later the next day, the double-decker took us to our next location. The bus was so tall that to pass through some of the lower underpasses, it pulled off of the road and expelled air from the shocks so it would fit. Once through, the bus pulled off of the road, and with the flip of a switch, re-filled the air shocks to raise up the bus.

When we visited Munich, two good-looking men bought us our first liter of beer, telling us that this was a town tradition to steal one of the heavy stoneware steins from the Hofbrau House. I had a huge purse. When I emptied the mug, I shoved it to the bottom of my purse before we left. Outside, I pulled out my souvenir to the laughter of our new friends as they escorted us to our hotel.

While in Munich, we saw the Rathaus-Glockenspiel, a giant cuckoo clock in the main square, as it performed its hourly ritual to the sound of beer garden music. Life-sized German figures popped out of the doors and danced in a circle until they retreated behind closed doors awaiting the strike of the next hour. The clock drew huge crowds, who cheered the opening and the closing of the doors as if the figures were living actors able to hear them.

One of the most disturbing yet meaningful events of that trip was our visit to the concentration camp in Dachau. We were first guided into a darkened auditorium to watch a German language movie, a movie for which, we were told, we wouldn't need an interpreter to understand. We didn't know what they meant until we saw the movie, a graphic depiction of the suffering of the camp's prisoners, showing footage of skeletal prisoners in striped uniforms, beatings, piles of broken corpses, mass graves. Even the most cynical smartasses among us cried in horror at the existence of such evil in the world.

After the movie, we walked through the camp, stunned. We sat on the tiny plywood bunkbeds that slept four people across. We went speechless as they led us into a gas chamber, closing the solid door behind us as we imagined the panic and screams of the people for whom this had been a reality. We stood at the lip of "the blood ditch," where tens of thousands had been slaughtered for refusing to comply, for being sick, or for being who they were—Jews, political prisoners, gay. We saw piles of human teeth that had been pulled post-mortem because they contained gold. We also were told about the inhuman experiments performed on pregnant women in labor as well as the elderly and the ill. The experience left me with a profound sorrow at how cruel humans can be. That experience didn't change me overnight into a different person, but it was always in the back of my mind, urging me to do better.

+ + +

When I graduated, I was shocked to receive a monetary award from a local women's group, but when I learned it was need-based, it made more sense. I figured I'd use it to pay for books when I started college.

Many of my friends were going away for college, but all I could manage was a contingent acceptance at Penn State Berks, the local campus of Pennsylvania State University. This meant that I would be living at home (certainly cheaper for my parents and me) and that I essentially would be starting college on academic probation. If I screwed up my grades, I was out.

When my friends started packing up to leave, I felt left out, as if I was the biggest loser of all time. I found it ironic that the same school system that just twelve years earlier named a reading group after me as the best reader in the first grade, now considered me (despite the award) a bad student. What was worse, I believed them. I couldn't really put it into words then, but now I know that being repeatedly raped for most of the year I was thirteen had robbed me of more than my virginity—it had robbed me of my childhood, my innocence, my sense of self. And in my shame, I felt that that was what I deserved.

CHAPTER 9

FALLING FOR THE MARLBORO MAN

I reluctantly started classes at Penn State Berks Campus just after Labor Day. Not only was I not crazy about living at home, I wasn't crazy about my major, Nutrition. Ever since my father's first heart attack, I had wanted to be a cardiologist, but my grades were so bad I couldn't even think about pre-med. Nutrition was medical adjacent and looked easy enough, so that's what I chose.

In the early days, I hung out with Jim, whom I knew from high school, and Bob, an older, more affluent student who drove a huge silver Mercedes and put on lavish parties. I dated Russ, from Irwin, Pennsylvania, for while, until he cheated on me with an underclassman I hated—at a party at my girlfriend's apartment no less. When I found out, I was devastated, but I wasn't putting up with that nonsense, and I broke up with him.

Then I met the man who would send my life on another detour.

While walking through the cafeteria one day, I noticed a table full of cute guys watching and pointing at me, laughing. I thought, *What, do I have ketchup on my face?* I think I actually rubbed my cheek. One of them, the best-looking one, so ruggedly handsome I dubbed him the Marlboro Man, stared at me more directly. I didn't know any of them, and because this was how Brent the rapist had begun his pursuit, I left through the closest door, more than slightly agitated.

This continued over the next week or so—most of the guys at the table laughing and pointing, while the Marlboro Man watched me intently. Finally one day, the Marlboro Man pushed away from the table and approached me. My heart picked up its beat, and I didn't know whether to run or talk to him. I talked to him. He introduced himself as Dennis, and invited me to sit at their table. He seemed nice enough, was very good looking, and I was a people pleaser who almost never said no to anyone. I followed Dennis back to the table and sat down in the chair someone had saved for me.

His friends were Keith, Bryan, and Joe. Once I sat with them for a while, I saw they weren't nearly as smug as they appeared. They explained why they laughed when I passed their table. They weren't laughing at me. They were laughing at Dennis's new nickname, "Tongue."

"Tongue?" I said.

"Because every time he sees you he gets tongue-tied," explained one of them. They all laughed, including Dennis.

At least they weren't laughing at me. After a few minutes, I remembered I had to get to class, and when I stood up to leave, Dennis followed me to the door. Without preamble, he asked me on a date for Saturday. I said, "Yes." I was on the rebound from Russ, and I wasn't going to turn down a date with this good-looking man.

On Saturday night we double dated with Keith and his girlfriend, Holly. We went to dinner at a restaurant I'd never been to, where the food and service were good, but the company left a lot to be desired. Keith was fine, a sensible and good looking, dark-haired guy, the slightest bit paunchy, but funny, with a dry sense of humor. He cracked us all up all dinner long.

Holly was another story, with her poorly dyed, bleached-blonde hair that fell in a disheveled mop to her shoulders, granny glasses she obsessively pushed up on her nose, and a shabby dress and ratty sweater. I couldn't tell whether she was dressing up or down. She was overbearing and talked non-stop, as if everything she had to say should be recorded for posterity. I knew we'd never be friends and wondered what Keith saw in her. *Is she that good in bed?* I thought, uncharitably.

Dennis himself was fairly quiet, listening to his friends chatter away, glancing at me to see how I was taking it all in. After dinner, Dennis walked me to my front door and gave me a quick kiss on the lips before I stepped inside. I thought the date had gone well. Dennis was nice, though I was surprised to find that he was six years older than I was. I usually dated older guys, but not that much older.

The next time I saw him, he asked me to go out on another date, and I accepted. Dennis asked me out a few more times after that, I said yes, and before long, we were exclusive. Over the course of our dates, he shared bits and pieces of his life. He was born and raised in the Lancaster, Pennsylvania area. His mom and dad were divorced, and his mom had moved to Berks County and remarried. His dad was a cop, working in the greater Lancaster area, but Dennis didn't talk about him much.

When I went to visit his mom and stepdad in Wyomissing Hills, an affluent suburb, I could see they were some degree of wealthy, but probably not as wealthy or important as Jo, his mom, wanted to be. She took me room by room to tell me all about the furnishings in the house, who she used as a decorator, which seamstress made her draperies, where they bought their expensive furniture, blah, blah, blah. She told me how to replace a roll of toilet paper properly, and how she and Doug (her husband) knew all the wealthiest democrats in the county. She quizzed me on which side of the plate the silverware went on. I listened respectfully—people pleaser!—all the while thinking, *Does it look like I give two shits?*

After we dated for a few months, Dennis asked me to marry him. I accepted before I really knew him. He seemed to be such a nice guy. He wanted to get married quickly. We jumped right in to planning the wedding, which was set for six months after the engagement.

When Jo found out, she insisted we have the wedding and reception at their place. Dennis and I both agreed, as it would save money, especially for my mom and dad. As the planning went on, however, it became the Jo show. She soon stopped even pretending to ask me what I thought, and made all the important decisions without me. This was too far even for me, the people pleaser. I shut that down and told Dennis I had picked a different venue.

He said he was fine with whatever I wanted for my special day, but I wonder. Soon after that, things changed between Dennis and me. For one thing, he was six years older than I was and still in college. For another, he had used heroin, with a needle, a fact I discovered when he told me about Woodstock and his life around that time. He was filmed for the documentary, and proudly pointed himself out when we watched the movie together. I didn't recognize the emaciated, disheveled, and mud-covered druggie in the video! He looked stoned out of his mind. And yes, I also used drugs, mostly pot and coke every once in a blue moon, but I drew a hard line at intravenous drugs.

I asked myself, *Why do you want to marry this guy again?* And the answer I came to was, *I don't. I don't love him anymore—if I ever did.* But then my next thought was, how was I going to tell Dennis and everybody else who was part of the wedding? By that time I had already asked my friends to be in the wedding, which was set for August 7, and we had purchased our gowns. We had also reserved and paid for the reception hall, and ordered the food, flowers, rings, cake, decorations, and everything else required for a wedding.

Could I disappoint all these people, and worse—cost them money they couldn't get back? I thought about it long and hard, and the answer was *No, I have to go through with this.* I'd rather suck it up and marry someone I didn't love than disappoint the people I did love.

At least my friends will still like me, and that's what I craved more than any drug: love. And I was willing to sell my soul for love. My mouth was only for eating, because I never spoke up for myself. I never had an opinion about anything. I just said what I thought others wanted to hear. And because I couldn't tell anybody about this—including myself until now—I felt helpless and alone.

Just after I decided to go through with it, I missed my period. *Oh, dear Lord, what am I going to do now?* I prayed. Two days later I took a blood test and received the verification by phone. I was torn by the news—happy because now I knew could have children; apprehensive because I was about to have a child with someone I didn't love.

I told Dennis that same day when he came to the house. I took him downstairs for privacy, then came right out with it. "Dennis, you're going to be a daddy!" I said.

He didn't say a word, but his face twisted red with anger.

"We are NOT going to have this child," he said, raising his voice.

"What do you mean?" I said. I had naively thought Dennis would be happy about the baby. *Isn't that why you got married?*

"I mean, you have to have an abortion!"

"An abortion?" I said. That had never crossed my mind. "Are you serious?"

"Of course I'm serious!" he barked. "I can't have a kid. That's not part of the plan. We'll go to Planned Parenthood as soon as we can get an appointment."

I was speechless. Abort our child? I never heard anything so cruel! *I'm so sorry, precious child,* I said to myself, rubbing my tummy.

Several long days later, Dennis drove me to Planned Parenthood on South Fourth Street in Reading. I was numb as the doctor examined me, trying not to cry. Dennis told her we wanted to schedule the abortion as soon as possible. Not that anyone was asking me what I wanted. Before we left the facility, we had a date and time for the abortion in Philadelphia. At that moment, I hated Dennis and what he was forcing me to do. How could he claim to be a Christian? But just as

I was helpless in the face of the wedding, I felt helpless to do anything else but what Dennis wanted.

"Don't worry, I'll take you to Philadelphia," he said.

The next few days were difficult to get through. I was throwing up with morning sickness, which lasted all day, and the rage I felt toward Dennis didn't help either. *Was I sick because I was pregnant or because of the pending abortion?*

The morning of the appointment was particularly bad. I was meeting Dennis in a parking lot near campus, but I could barely walk with the nausea, let alone drive. At least Dennis was driving the rest of the way to Philadelphia. I forced myself to stand tall and cheerfully holler "Good-bye" so my parents wouldn't suspect anything was wrong. I could never have told them I was aborting their grandchild. I blasted the air conditioning in the car, hoping the cold air might help.

I was surprised that Dennis wasn't waiting for me in the parking lot, but I pulled into a shady space, thrilled to be able to rest. I closed my eyes, but no Dennis. It was an hour and a half drive, and we had to leave soon to be on time. I hoped everything was okay. He was usually prompt when we met up. I pushed it as close to the cut off as I could, and it struck me that he wasn't coming. He had blown me off. "That son of a bitch," I said, hitting the gas pedal hard. I turned on the radio and cried most of the way to the facility.

I entered the building dry heaving and fiddling with my ring. A pleasant woman greeted me and took me back to get changed, then led me into a cold exam room. I wanted to be anywhere else but there. My heart pounded and my throat went dry. I spoke in croaks and mumbles. Then the doctor came in and introduced himself in a monotone with zero personal warmth. Apparently, I wasn't the only one who didn't want to be there.

I was helped onto the exam table, my feet put in the stirrups, a noisy machine turned on. I closed my eyes and sobbed as he inserted the suction device through my cervix and moved it around my uterus. I heard the body parts slapping through the tube, and I cried even harder. Just when I thought I couldn't take it anymore, someone turned off the equipment and the doctor pulled out the tube.

I was relieved it was over, but I trembled in pain and guilt at the end of a precious life. I don't remember getting dressed or getting in the car, but I do remember sobbing violently all the way home. Part of me had died with the fetus, and I didn't know how I'd come back from that.

I don't remember much about the aftermath with Dennis. I know we had a huge fight about him leaving me high and dry, but out of self-preservation, I've repressed most of the details.

A few awful, short weeks later was our wedding day, and I dreaded the thought of it. I wasn't feeling very festive, for one thing, still bleeding and cramping from the abortion. And certainly, Dennis's blowing off the abortion appointment didn't make me want to marry him more.

It was a rainy, cold August morning when I opened my eyes. *Fitting weather*, I thought. "Happy is the bride that has rain on her special day!" Mom said when I went upstairs. *What Bullshit!* But to Mom I smiled and nodded. I had to put on a good show. No one could know how I really felt.

I did my own makeup at home, then met the girls at the church to get dressed: Maxine, my maid of honor; Valerie, Peggy, Eileen, Kim, Joy, Shelley, and Dennis's step sisters, Sandy and Eileen, my bridesmaids; and my niece Heidi, the flower girl. The guys had arrived as well. Heidi's brother Michael was the ring bearer, and my brothers Kenny and Kevin were ushers. The flowers had already been delivered and arranged. The archway looked beautiful, too beautiful for this sad wedding.

We had the use of one of the basement rooms. We heard people moving around upstairs, meaning the guests were arriving. We could just barely hear Lynn tuning her acoustic guitar and strumming a few chords to warm up. Lynn was the friend I had hired to play at the wedding. I couldn't wait to hear her beautiful voice sing the Wedding Song, just about the only thing I was looking forward to. I prayed that someone would come downstairs and tell me Dennis had called the church to call off the wedding, that he wasn't showing up.

No such luck. We got the word to head upstairs and after checking myself in the mirror one last time, I grabbed Dad's hand and said, "Are you ready?"

"I'm ready," he said, squeezing my hand. Couldn't he see into my soul that marrying Dennis was the last thing I wanted to do? Couldn't he swoop in in his white tuxedo and rescue his little girl? No, how could he? The organ had launched into a slow processional that sounded like a funeral march. I gave him a big, reassuring, fake smile, and we headed upstairs.

My attendants lined up in the vestibule as we had practiced the night before. One by one, the girls headed down the aisle, until it was time for Dad and me. I kept my head down for the first few steps, then raised it and found Dennis waiting with his groomsmen at the altar. He had gotten a perm! It looked awful, artificial, like he had thrown on a wig! What was he thinking? He no longer looked like the Marlboro man. More like Bozo the clown.

Midway through the service, the pastor paused so Lynn could sing the Wedding Song, the one made popular by Peter, Paul, and Mary. It was the highlight of the ceremony, the only part I enjoyed. She sang it perfectly, and my eyes filled with tears. "Whenever two or more of you are gathered in his name, there is love." *If only*, I thought.

I spent more time at the reception with my friends than Dennis, drinking and dancing with each other like girls do. Somewhere around nine, I heard a commotion. Dennis's mom was screaming at my brother Kevin. She was right up in his face, the poster child for spitting mad. Someone snapped on the overhead lights, and that was that, the reception was over. Embarrassed guests left abruptly, and my friends carried the gifts to the cars.

I never learned what the fight was about, exactly. It was inevitable that she would cause a scene, though, since I had cut her out of the planning and this brought the attention back to her. I was so angry that when Dennis told me he was going to say goodbye to her and Doug, I refused to join him and told him his family was no longer invited to the brunch at my parents' house the next day. I was so embarrassed in front of my girlfriends that I never contacted any of them who were there again, except Shelley.

I've blocked out so much about that day (and that marriage) that I can't remember where we spent our wedding night. I do remember that we fought about his mother's scene and the rest of the night we seethed silently in anger and hatred. I know that we did not consummate the marriage that night, since I was still bleeding from the abortion. If he had come anywhere near me, I might have neutered him then and there. I do remember going to my parents' house to open our wedding presents the following day, but only my family was invited. Then in the mid-afternoon we got into my copper-colored Plymouth Arrow for the six-hour trip to Williamsburg, Virginia.

I must have swum in the pool in Williamsburg. I know this because many years later I found a colored snapshot of me in a two-piece, mint green swimsuit sitting at the edge of the pool, legs in the water. The young woman in the photo was heavy with the weight of it all. The picture took me back and I remember thinking at the time, why didn't I have the courage to say no? I promised myself then and there, August 9, 1976, while sitting at the edge of the pool, alone, that I would never let anything like this happen again. On impulse years later I tore the picture into tiny pieces and sprinkled it in a waste basket. I never wanted to see myself like that again.

We left for Florida the following morning, and the remainder of the honeymoon was uneventful. We basked in the sun all day, had a later dinner, and then went off to bed exhausted. I'm sure he was clueless about how I really felt. We took two days to drive back to Pennsylvania, fighting only a little about his mother.

Dennis moved in to my apartment in my parents' basement. We had both decided not to return to college in September. Dennis got a sales position, and I became a proof consultant at a photography studio. Because I worked alone at the studio, when I least expected it, I had flashbacks to the abortion—me on the exam table, in stirrups, forced to listen to all those suction sounds that still haunted me! I didn't know how to get these sights and sounds out of my head. It scared me, and I didn't have a single person to talk to.

Married life was like acting in a play. Like many survivors of sexual assault, I became adept at faking it, putting on a show of normal. I did my best to make Dennis believe I loved him. I cooked for him, cleaned for him, washed his clothing, and dear God, did my wifely duties and had the blandest of bland sex with him—missionary style, no foreplay, no oral sex. He only took care of his own needs, and those very quickly, which became part of the appeal, since I felt no pleasure. The faster the better.

To help me through it, while I lay there beneath his grunting desire I designed large hotels with the most ornate features in the style of medieval castles, including heavy dark tapestries on the walls and beautiful draperies everywhere. I picked out the colors, I picked out the texture. It was so real to me I could feel the rough weave of the tapestries, the smoothness of the drapes, the smell of the paint as I redid each room, sometimes in soft, soothing colors, other times in colors that were bright and electrifying. All my castles had spiral stairs, window turrets, ornate doors, and the most thick and luxurious wall hangings to keep the chill down and flank the windows. I probably redecorated a million rooms while I was married to Dennis.

I also turned back to alcohol to help me through these ordeals. If I sensed Dennis was in the mood, I had a few drinks beforehand. Did other wives feel like I did? Like my life was over at nineteen? Like Kim had disappeared into this stranger called Dennis's wife? I didn't have anyone to talk to about it—certainly not Mom. I didn't want to burden her. I was trapped in a living nightmare. What had I been thinking? All I could do was pray to my Lord for grace and deliverance.

Once we were married, Dennis began acting strangely. Most evenings when he got home from work, he already smelled of alcohol, but when I asked him about it, he snarled, "Mind your own business!". If that wasn't bad enough, he got fired every couple of weeks from whatever job he managed to get. He must have been drinking the day away instead of working.

And the nights. Some nights he didn't come home until one or two in the morning. His favorite bar was Your Place Bar and Restaurant. I had reason to suspect he was sleeping with the blonde barmaid he talked about too much.

I put up with it, put up with it, put up with it, until I couldn't. One night he didn't come home until mid-morning the next day. I was alone in our apartment. Toby, my large, black dog was upstairs when Dennis opened the door and stumbled inside. I was in the kitchen. I turned to him and said, "Where in the hell have you been all night?"

"It's none of your fucking business where I've been."

"Excuse me, you're a married man and married men sleep in their own homes with their wife!"

At that, he ran at me and tackled me to the concrete floor, then held me down, grabbing my neck between his hands and squeezing until I couldn't breathe. He banged my head on the floor over and over again. I saw stars each time, and I grew dizzy and panicky from lack of air. I clawed at his clenched hands, but they squeezed even tighter around my throat. *He's going to kill me*, I thought. *He's going to kill me. At least the nightmare will be over.*

And just when I was about to give up and let go, I heard Mom's voice. "What the hell are you doing to my daughter?" Dennis released my throat, and I took a hit of air that was better than any joint I had ever smoked. "Get off her now and get the fuck out of my house—and don't come back!" Mom almost never raised her voice, but when she did, watch out. Threaten her family, and she turned into a she-wolf.

Dennis jumped to his feet, strutted to the door to show he wasn't scared of her, then sneered before he walked out of our tiny apartment for the last time.

Mom crouched at my side on the floor as I sat up, breathing hard, my head sore and pounding. Toby pranced down the steps and nuzzled my hand. I pushed myself from the floor, and went into the bathroom where the illuminated mirror revealed the handprints around my neck. I cried as I rubbed the back of my head, telling Mom between sobs, "I never want him back here, Mom. I was NEVER in love with that monster. I never wanted to marry him, but I didn't know how to tell you after all that money you put into it."

"Kim, I never liked Dennis, and neither did Dad or Eugene. We never wanted you to marry him either, but we thought you were happy. That's why we never said anything."

"I was quite the actress. Sorry, Mom."

"We couldn't have cared less about the money. You're more important than any money we spent. Heck, we would have thrown a party to celebrate that you didn't marry him!"

We laughed and hugged and cried. Mom came through for me again that night.

Over the next few days, I conferred with my parents about what to do. Together we decided I should see an attorney to start the divorce. I made an appointment with an attorney Dad knew from high school. The attorney suggested that he send a letter to Dennis to request temporary alimony since Dennis had a better job than I did. I agreed and he sent the letter.

About a week after my appointment with the attorney, I was working one evening at the photography studio. I had picked up the next set of proofs and casually looked through each picture, then raised my head to think about them. And there was Dennis standing on the other side of the counter. The second we made eye contact, he spewed out a string of nasty comments, then took a swing at my face. I stepped back and dodged the punch.

"You'll never get another cent out of me, bitch," he snarled, then stormed out the door. *Okay*, I thought. *That wasn't too bad. Nothing I can't handle.*

The remainder of the night was uneventful but busy. I showed proofs to a number of customers and helped them pick the ones they wanted blown up and framed. At the end of the night, Donna, the photographer, and I locked up, and walked toward our cars.

My windshield was shattered. The closer I got to the car, the more obvious the damage became. You could still see where his fist hit the wind shield. Shards of glass covered the seats, making it impossible to drive. I found a note and a one-dollar bill shoved in the door handle. It read, "This is all the money you'll ever get from me!"

Donna and I went back inside to call the police, a tow truck, and my parents. "I can't stand that man," I said to Donna. She looked at me as if to say, *Yeah, I got that.*

I got in touch with my attorney, and we filed a restraining order. What a nightmare, like I was living in a trashy novel. At twenty years old, I felt like such a failure. I had let so many people down, but most of all myself.

Since I was avoiding all my friends who had been at the wedding, I asked Donna if she felt like a drink one day after work, and she said, "Sure." We tried Johnny's Café in Shillington. After we ordered the first round, I saw someone else I knew there—Barb and her husband, Mike. They had graduated with my brother Kevin. They invited us to their table, where we had a few more drinks and a lot of laughs. They told me some things about Kevin he probably didn't want me to know. It was the first time in a long while I forgot about Dennis and what a loser I was. As the night ended, we swapped information and made plans to get back together. I had found a new friend, one who would change my life forever.

CHAPTER 10

SWEET REVENGE

About two weeks later, on a rainy, gloomy day, Mom hollered down the stairs to let me know two men were at the door asking to speak to me. "They look official," she added.

Official? I wondered. When I met them in the living room, I saw what she meant. They both wore beige trench coats. When they saw me, they reached inside their coats to reveal their FBI badges. *What the heck?*

They must have seen the question in my face, so they jumped right into it. "Are you Kim Goodling, married to Dennis Goodling?" asked one of them.

"Ye-es," I said. "But we're getting a divorce. What's he done?"

"That's what you can help us with," said the other. "We want to question him about a rape, but we need you to identify his car. Will you come with us?"

I wasn't really surprised. They gave me the outline of what had happened. He had—allegedly—taken a young girl at knifepoint from a bus stop, held her hostage all day, raped her multiple times, and then, when school was over, dropped her off at the bus stop. The girl had identified items in a blue station wagon they believed was parked at Your Place.

"If you verify that's his car, he's going to jail."

"I'd be happy to. Give me a sec." I went and got my things, then followed them through the rain to their unmarked car with its telltale antenna. I didn't want to waste any time.

As we drove to Your Place in silence, a thousand things ran through my head. Has he done this before? Was he doing it while we lived together? Could I have stopped him somehow? Oh, my goodness, I realized, horrified. I remembered something his parents had told me early on. His step-sister, Debbie, who was legally blind from birth, had been raped just before I knew them by an intruder who knew how to get in the house and knew exactly where to find her. The weird thing was, Dennis's mom had told me, their mean old poodle, Charlie, who barked maniacally at strangers, hadn't made a sound. *It must have been him!* I gasped. *Dennis had raped his blind stepsister.*

Should I say something? I wondered. It took me less than a second to speak up. "Do you know about the sister's rape?" I asked.

The agent in the passenger's seat looked back at me and said, "No, we do not."

"Less than a year ago, Dennis's blind stepsister was raped in their home in Wyomissing Hills," I recounted. "They could never solve the crime. The dog never barked, I was told, though he went crazy with strangers."

The agents looked at each other, then looked back at me. "Well, that certainly adds fuel to the fire," the same agent said.

When we pulled into the parking lot, there it was, plain as day, Dennis's blue station wagon. He must have been sitting at the bar, drinking. We had to go through the protocol, though. They had me get out of their car and examine Dennis's car more closely. I looked inside the rear windows, then said, "Yes, absolutely. This is Dennis's car."

"Okay. Thank you, Ma'am. We'll take you home, then make the arrest."

"Can I watch?" I said.

He looked at me quizzically, then said, "That bad?"

I nodded.

"I'm afraid not," the agent said. "For your safety."

I was disappointed—I wanted to see him in handcuffs—but I understood.

They sped back to my parents' house, and left the driveway before I opened the door. Mom and Dad were in the living room, waiting for me.

"Can you believe this?" I said when I saw them. I told them I had wanted to stay for the arrest, but the agents wouldn't let me.

"The CB Radio!" Dad said. "We can listen to the chatter."

I laughed. "I'll get the beer."

After I tapped three beers, I met Mom and Dad in the office, where we cheered Dennis's arrest. This might seem ghoulish, but we were giddy with relief. Since Mom had kicked him out, he had called her regularly, claiming he had kidnapped me and describing in detail how he planned to hurt me. It was never true, Mom would find out when I walked through the door later. But Mom never knew when he might make good on his threat.

"It's over," I said. "His freedom just ended."

I wasn't asked to testify. Once the FBI agents took me home, I never heard from them again. We learned from the newspaper that Dennis was found guilty and sent to Graterford State Prison with a five-year sentence. Five years wasn't long enough for me, but it was better than nothing. When he got out, he married the daughter of the jail chaplain, and they lived in the greater Reading area and had a daughter, but that marriage ended in divorce as well.

I recently found out that Rod has kept tabs on Dennis. I know that Dennis is married to a third wife and lives somewhere in Missouri. His legal record shows only a DUI. A friend who worked in the Arizona prison system told me he must have accepted a plea deal—that would be the only way for his record to be expunged. People get longer sentences for possession of marijuana.

To this day, I haven't seen him again. Sometimes God does answer your prayers.

PART III

LIFE REBOOTED

No matter how hard the past is,
you can always begin again.

—Jack Kornfield

CHAPTER 11

....

BASEBALL WITH BARB

Since after my disaster of a wedding I had pushed away many of my old friends, I spent more time with Barb. We'd go out for drinks and chat on the phone. I'm a social person, with the gift of making friends. I have always had good friends.

One evening over drinks, Barb asked if I'd go with her to her husband's softball game the next night. "It's so boring. I could use someone to talk to."

"Sure," I said. "I've got nothing else going on. I'll come over after work."

I rode with Barb and Mike, her husband, to the game. Barb and I sat in the bleachers and talked through the whole game, occasionally clapping when someone had a good hit or scored a run. Barb and I were getting to know each other. Her mom was a secretary at the middle school, and when I was in school, she had always been nice to me. After the game, we went to the team bar, and I got to know some of the guys and their wives and girlfriends. Most of the guys on the team had graduated from Governor Mifflin, my high school, so I already knew many of them. It was a good night, something new and different.

Barb soon asked me to go to all of the games, and I said, "Sure, why not, as long as I don't have to work." They typically played three games a week, and if I couldn't make the game, I met them at the bar.

The first night I couldn't attend I met Barb afterwards. "Wait until you hear what happened to me at the game," Barb said, rolling her eyes.

"This must be good," I said.

"Do you know who Robin is?"

"No clue."

"Well, this Robin sat down next to me and asked if I was bringing you to the games to watch her fiancé pitch."

"Her fiancé?"

"Rod. Rod Shipe. The pitcher."

"Still no clue. That's bizarre! Are they here now?"

"I don't see them."

"Next game, point them out."

"He's a nice guy, but she's a bit flighty, a motormouth. Bleached blonde. Been around the block a few times."

When I finally met Robin, it wasn't at a game. Barb and I and some others were at Johnny's Café. Barb pulled me aside and said, "There's Robin on the far side of the bar. I'll introduce you."

We walked over, and Barb started up a conversation. Then Barb turned and said, "Robin, I'd like you to meet my girlfriend, Kim."

"Hi, nice to meet you," I said to be polite, but I was not impressed. She had a foul mouth. Everything was fucking this or bullshit that, and I assumed her fiancé, Rod, of whom she was so possessive, was the same.

I still went to the games with Barb and Mike to keep Barb company. Then came the last game of the summer on a very warm evening. We ended up at Johnny's Café as usual. Rod was there without Robin, and he ended up sitting next to me at the bar, with Barb and Mike on my other side. Now that I actually talked with Rod, I saw he wasn't like Robin at all, though I did wonder why such a smart, thoughtful, and, yes, good-looking guy was with a woman like that!

When the bar closed at two, Rod suggested we all go Ocean City, New Jersey, and we were just tipsy enough to agree. Rod followed me home so I could get my swimsuit, a beach towel, a change of clothes, and some cash and let my mom know where we were going. I didn't have cash and neither did Mom, but she had just rolled her jar of quarters and gave me a roll: $20.00.

We met up with Barb and Mike. Barb had not had as much to drink as the three of us, so she agreed to drive, with one requirement. "Kim needs to sit up front to help with directions."

We talked for a bit once we were on our way, but soon the three passengers fell sound asleep. At one point, Barb called my name and shook me. "Kim, what's our exit?"

"Cantaloupe," I mumbled, opening my eyes for a second before falling back to sleep.

Barb laughed. "Cantaloupe? That's not an exit." She was on her own.

She got us there, though! As she crossed the last bridge onto the barrier island of Ocean City, then pulled into an empty space along the beach, she called out. "Everyone wake up! We're here!"

"Already?" I said sleepily.

"No thanks to you. You told me to get off at cantaloupe!"

"I did? I don't remember that!"

We laughed ourselves awake, then made our way to the beach, where we spread out our blankets. I found a space between Barb and Rod. Mike was on the other side of his wife. It didn't take us long to fall asleep, that snug, cozy, delicious kind of sleep you can only get on a beach in the late summer sun amidst the smell of salt water and French fries. We didn't wake until mid-day hunger set in.

"Anyone want to head to the Anchorage Inn for lunch?" asked Rod.

We all agreed and packed up for the day.

We took a short car ride back to the mainland to get to the Anchorage Inn in Somers Point, where we enjoyed lunch and a few cold drafts. I found Rod to be nice and extremely polite, always opening my car door and helping me with my seat at restaurants. He was easy to talk to. He told me that he was several credits away from getting his Masters in Clinical Psychology. We discussed some case studies, without naming names, of course. He had a way of making everything funny, whether the patients he was studying or the people in the restaurant with us, and he kept us all laughing. I felt lighter than I had in a very long time, exhilarated.

But all good things have to end, and we made our way back to real life. Rod and I didn't make plans, but I knew I'd see him again even with the end of softball season, once he broke off his engagement. I had that feeling. I just had to be content to wait on the Lord's time.

CHAPTER 12

GOOD THINGS COME TO THOSE WHO WAIT

Our Ocean City lark had been at the end of August. Rod didn't return to our nightly hangout until the night of my twenty-second birthday, October 14, 1978. How he knew it was my birthday is still a mystery; I assume Barb and Mike had something to do with it, but no one ever confirmed or denied. He even brought me a present—white gold hoop earrings—a pleasant surprise since it had been so long since I had seen him. I was feeling good. I had a new job I liked—working with the most severely disabled children in the county. This was icing on the cake.

We talked and drank and laughed, then some time during the night he popped the question. (No, not *that* question. Not yet, anyway.) "Will you go on a date with me?"

"Not if you're engaged," I said. I had standards, and I wanted him to understand that.

"I broke it off with Robin," he said.

I watched his face as he said this to make sure it wasn't a line. It wasn't a line. "Okay, then. Yes." I smiled. Things were looking up.

"How about the Hershey Bears game on *my* birthday?"

The Hershey Bears are team in the American Hockey League. His birthday was just two weeks after mine, October 30.

"Sounds great!" I said. "I've never been to a Bears game."

We talked and laughed the rest of the night. I told him about my new job and how much I enjoyed working with disabled children, how rewarding I found it. I always liked helping people. He told me he had a seven-year-old son named Jason. Jason lived in Mohnton with his mom and stepdad. I told him I was going through a nasty divorce of my own which would be finalized soon. He was easy to talk to, warm and open and a good listener. We could talk about almost anything. By the end of the night, we felt we had known each other for years.

The next week was busy at work, and when it was that busy, I stayed home at night and watched TV. At work I had become friends with Chris, another teacher. In passing she told me about Laura, a fortune teller she had been seeing for quite some time. She described Laura as a different kind of fortune teller, an older woman who kept a Bible in front of her during the reading. And everything she told Chris had come true!

I told Chris I didn't believe in that sort of nonsense. That they got the information from research or by chitchat before the reading, or the observations were so open ended they could apply to anyone. Chris was convinced she was the real deal and challenged me to make an appointment. Of course, I was a cocky twenty-two year old. I picked up the phone and called Laura at her home, a few miles away in Kenhorst, and she said, "Why don't you come over today after you finish work?" She wouldn't have the time to look up anything about me, and I'd be able to tell Chris she was full of it.

Laura's house was easy to find. She was hunched over, with short grey hair, and wore a house dress over her pudgy body. We sat at a large dining room table, she at the head with a Bible in front of her, me at her right. Around the house were plastic flower arrangements of harvest gold, olive green, and burnt orange on top of doilies. She asked if I brought something to write on. I shook my head. She retrieved a stack of paper towels from the kitchen, the brown ones you might find in a school restroom. I chuckled to myself about this quirky woman. *Harmless enough*, I thought. *I'll humor her.*

I'm glad I wrote everything down and kept those paper towels all these years.

She told me she had been fiddling with the Bible as we chatted, and she turned to the same page three times. There must be a message for me there. She summed it up for me. On the third day after childbirth I should do nothing because that's when my organs would be go back into place. If I overdid things, my organs would never be the same! Then she began spouting information so fast I could barely keep up. Sometimes I'd try to slow her down with a question or ask for her to repeat what she said.

Here is the gist of what I wrote down: "Pretty soon you are going to have a date with a man who is a lot taller than you, either this fall or in the spring. I see him wearing a corduroy blazer as he stands at your front door. That's the man you are going to marry. You will have a short engagement and get married relatively soon. Your life with this man will be very similar to your life before 1967. Does that make sense to you?"

"Yes, it does. That's when my dad came back from Vietnam, and he left the Army a year later due to medical issues. Things went downhill after that."

"The two of you are going to have two children, a boy and a girl. Your son will eventually have two children, both girls, and your daughter will have three children, two girls and a boy. You are going to live to a ripe old age, and you will get to see your grandchildren and even your great grandchildren. Soon after this first date, you will fly somewhere with this man, possibly to a family event. He will meet your family.

It will be like a short vacation for the two of you. Your family will like him very much. You will travel many other places together.

"Your father did a lot of marching and because of this, he has suffered many health issues. His mother thanks you for something you did at her grave. You are going to go to school and change your career, and when this happens, you'll think of me! You aren't really aware of this yet, but you are a healer, and you will heal many people over the course of your life. If you burn candles, always burn orange candles. You have the most beautiful and colorful aura, very unique."

Then she stopped the reading itself and chatted about her own life, how her husband had died and left her alone.

Suddenly, I realized the time and said I had to get going. Before I did, though, I asked, "Do you see anything bad in my life?"

She paused and turned her head as if she was listening. "No, there's nothing I see that's bad in your life."

Relieved, I gathered the many paper towels and thanked Laura for the reading. The fee was twenty dollars, which I had already left on the table.

I headed toward the door when she said, "On your way home, stop and play the lottery with these three numbers: 067, boxed and straight. It will only cost a few dollars. I just had a premonition that my husband's favorite numbers are going to win the Pick Three tonight."

"All right," I said. "But I better get going. It's almost drawing time."

"Come back and see me again," she called out as I closed the door behind me.

On the drive home, I stopped at the corner store and bought a lottery ticket with those numbers. As I drove home, I thought about everything Laura had told me. What was I going to tell Chris tomorrow? Laura did seem to know some things about me.

I opened the front door just minutes before the seven o'clock drawing and turned on the TV, clutching the ticket. The numbers were 0, 6, 8! "Damn, off by one," I told my mother. "Good thing I didn't waste more money."

The next day at work, Chris wanted to know all the details of my reading. As soon as we had a free minute, I pulled the folded paper towels out of my purse.

"You're getting married soon? You aren't even dating anyone."

"I know," I said. I told her about the lottery and what she had said about my father. "I think I believe her. She has a gift."

"Everything Laura told me came true," Chris said. "I wish I could do that."

"Not me," I said. "I'm good just the way God made me!"

On Monday, October 30, I had my first official date with Rod. I had never been to a professional hockey game, and I was excited to see Rod again. We were going out for dinner after the game.

I was dressed to the nines and my makeup was perfect. My long, dark brown hair looked pretty against a pale pink blouse, and I had bought a new pair of blue jeans for the occasion. I grabbed a jacket at the last minute against the cool air of the hockey arena.

I was the only one home when the doorbell rang. When I opened the door, I saw a six-foot, six-inch young man in a tan corduroy blazer, just as Laura had described a few days earlier. *Is he really going to be my husband?* I mused as I stepped onto the front porch.

We had seats at ice level and saw a few fights right in front of us. Rod told me that was half the fun, and he was right. Afterwards, we had a great dinner at a nice steakhouse, with a carafe of wine and ice cream for dessert. Before the end of the night, he asked for another date, and I accepted. Who could fight fate? I didn't tell him about Laura's prediction that someday I'd be Mrs. Kim Shipe. I didn't want to scare him away.

We got along well and continued to go out regularly. We often double dated with Barb and Mike. Barb was the only other person who knew about Laura's prediction.

As we spent more time together, I met his family and got to know more about him—his seven-year-old son Jason; Rod's mom, Joann, and his stepdad, Johnny; his stepbrothers Jack and Jeff, who were both in high school; and his grandparents, Ma and Pa. They all lived in the same house. Rod was especially close to his grandparents. He told me his grandma was more like a mom to him than his own mom.

Jason lived only a few miles away from my parents' house, so I got to see him with Rod a fair amount. Since we didn't want to antagonize Jason's mother, we always picked him up and dropped him off on time. I loved to watch Rod and Jason together because of the tender way Rod cared for him. Jason was also going to be tall when he grew up. He had boney knees and long slender legs, and he frequently tripped over his large feet when he walked. Rod often played basketball with him, and they always worked on the fundamentals before they played a game. They loved to watch action movies together during which Joann, Rod's mom, made them each a large bowl of buttered popcorn. Watching Rod in the daddy role told me he would be a good father to our children someday, but I didn't let on I was thinking that far ahead.

Mom and Dad drove to Michigan to visit my brother, Kevin, near Detroit. Kevin had gotten a job there after graduating from Penn State with a degree in architectural engineering, the same major as our older brother, Kenny. They planned to stay through Thanksgiving.

After my parents left, I invited Rod for Friday dinner. My parents knew all about it—after all, I had already been married once. I went to the Shillington Farmer's Market to shop for fresh meat and vegetables. I chose thick cut pork chops stuffed with Pennsylvania Dutch potato stuffing, which the butcher explained how to cook. When the night arrived, I followed the instructions to a T and also prepared a Caesar salad and broccoli au gratin while they were baking.

Rod arrived on time, and the house smelled of the delicious meal. He said he was hungry, so we sat down right away. I poured the wine, and we dug in. He ate everything I put in front of him, and had seconds as well. He had told me once that key lime pie was his favorite, so

I served that for dessert. When we finished, he pushed back from the table and told me that was the best dinner he'd ever had. Always the charmer. Although I was a little nervous, I had enjoyed it too.

That night he slept over. I hadn't expected that to happen, but I had made the bed with new sheets and a bedspread just in case. The next morning, we enjoyed coffee and breakfast. He said he had a few errands to run, but then he'd return. When he returned, he brought some clothes and hung them in my closet. I was surprised—pleasantly—when he said he was staying the whole weekend. I thought he'd leave on Sunday, but he surprised me again by staying.

Monday morning, we both got up for work and Rod said he'd be back again that night. Apparently he wasn't sick of me yet. Each evening that week he returned with more clothes to add to the closet. On one of my parents' calls, they said, "Why don't you and Rod fly up for Thanksgiving?" Rod said, "Sure," and we booked our flights. Another one of Laura's predictions had come true.

This was an important trip for me. I hadn't made such a good choice the first time around, and though I was smitten with Rod, I wanted my family's take on him.

Whenever we walked together, Rod held my hand, and that's how we met Kevin and our parents at the gate. It was my first time visiting Kevin since his graduation. He's the type A engineer. His apartment was well-organized and tidy, with his dishes spaced perfectly on the shelves and his utensils in alignment. Even his desk was clean and clear, with every one of his pencils and pens lined up in a special trough. Ever the little sister, I wondered, *What would happen if I messed everything up?*

I helped Mom prepare the turkey and the typical sides and pies—mashed potatoes, yams, green bean casserole, pumpkin pie. Over dinner, which was delicious, we laughed, joked, and talked about everything under the sun. Rod was quickly comfortable with my family, and they enjoyed him as well. After we pitched in with the clean up, Rod and I fell asleep in front of the TV. When we woke up, everyone except Dad played cards. I warned Mom not to help Kevin win like she used to.

"Did she really do that?" Rod asked.

"You bet she did. Kevin used to get so angry when he didn't win, Mom helped him out."

"Mom helped her win more than me," Kevin protested.

"Did not," I said in true sister style. "No one wanted to be around you when you lost."

"Tonight I'm going to kick your butt without any help!" he said, all in good fun.

Before we left on Sunday, I pulled Mom and my brother aside separately to ask them what they thought of Rod. They both really liked him. *Good*, I thought. By then, I was pretty sure Laura's prediction was going to come true.

Once we got back home after the holiday, Rod began to drop hints about the M-word—marriage. I acted surprised but I really wasn't— Laura was on the money again. *Wait until I tell Chris!*

We decided that since we were both married before, we didn't want a big wedding, just something small and intimate with family and close friends.

....

CHAPTER 13

THIS ONE'S A KEEPER

We were shooting for a January date, but as Christmas approached, we got so busy we didn't give ourselves enough time to plan a wedding, so we decided February would be fine. However, with each successive month, we put it off to the next month. And by we, I mean Rod.

Finally, it was March, and we still didn't have a date. I had a serious talk with Rod. "Do you really want to get married?" I asked.

"Yes, I do," Rod said.

"Then why do you keep pushing out the date?"

"We just never take the time to look at a calendar," Rod said.

"I think you have cold feet."

"That's not true. Get a calendar and we'll pick a date in April."

I grabbed the calendar from the kitchen. "Here's the April calendar." I handed it to him. "What date?"

Rod examined the calendar, placed his finger on one of the squares. "How about April 21?"

"That works for me. But I want you to understand, if we don't get married on April 21, I'm moving to California to live with Shelley!

I always wanted to live in California, and if we don't get married, when else would I do it?"

Rod looked at me as if to say, *really?* But I didn't back down.

I had already asked Barb to be my Matron of Honor. She had introduced us after all. My niece, Heidi, agreed to be our flower girl, and Rod's son our ring bearer. Byron, whom Rod had been living with when we met, would be Best Man. We chose the church Rod had attended with his grandparents when he lived with them, in Hamburg, Pennsylvania. We met with the pastor to finalize the details.

After I visited several bridal stores, I opted not to wear a typical wedding dress. I found the perfect dress for me in Donnecker's Dress Store, in Denver, Pennsylvania. It was a floor length, straight-line gown of the palest slate blue with a cream-colored short jacket, a single tie in front, and stitching that matched the dress. Rod found a nice suit to match. It had a white background with the smallest plaid pattern in slate blue and medium grey and a matching vest. Underneath he'd wear a crisp white shirt.

Nothing could stop us now. The forecast was perfect, with no rain in sight, a sunny, warm day with temperatures in the upper seventies. I woke up extra early to make sure everything was ready for the wedding and the reception, which would be at my parents' home, where guests could hang out inside or outside. We had plenty of food and snacks, beer on draft, and the most delicious cake with butter cream icing.

While I dealt with last minute logistics, Rod came to me and said out of the blue, "I love you, Kim."

"I love you more!" I said.

He walked over, bent down and kissed me on my lips before holding me briefly. Rod just melted me. He was so sensitive and loved to be close to me. He even held me in his arms when we slept.

Barb and I got dressed together. When she put her dress on, she looked down at her chest in horror. Her nipples showed through the pale yellow gown. We looked at each other as if to say, "What now?"

"Do you have any Band-Aids?" Barb asked.

"Will that work?"

"We better find out."

I brought her the Band-Aids, and she tried them out. They worked! Crisis averted. We giggled the whole time she helped me dress. For the final touch, she tucked sprigs of baby's breath in my hair, then helped me finish my makeup.

My niece, Heidi, the flower girl arrived around noon, dressed and ready for the wedding, looking adorable in the pale-yellow, floor length-dress. Rod was going to bring his son, Jason, the ring bearer, directly to the church.

Our wedding was set for two with the reception right after. We were going to leave at seven for our honeymoon on Chincoteague Island, Virginia.

We arrived at the church before the guys and waited in the basement. Within a few minutes, Jason joined us. Just before we were supposed to head upstairs, I noticed that Jason had dried mustard around his mouth. They had stopped for hot dogs on the way to the church! I wiped it off with a tissue, shaking my head.

And then it happened. We were called upstairs, and I married the most wonderful man in the world.

The church was a beautiful brownstone with a bright red front door and stained-glass windows of scenes from the Bible. My favorite was Jesus kneeling in prayer in Gethsemane. The pews were arranged like an amphitheater, wrapping around the altar where Rod stood tall. He was smiling broadly as I walked down the aisle with my arm looped in Dad's. I don't remember much of the ceremony. My head was in the clouds, and I was smiling a mile wide. We exchanged our vows and our rings, said our *I do's*, kissed, and we were husband and wife! I couldn't have been happier.

After the ceremony, we took pictures inside the church, outside the church, and across the street in the schoolyard next to the three-tiered fountain, then headed to Mom and Dad's in Shillington for the reception.

We enjoyed our reception—drinking and eating with the people who meant the most to us. When it came time to leave at seven, Rod asked, "Are you ready to go?"

"Let's stay longer," I said. "I'm having so much fun!"

We finally tore ourselves away at nine, since we had a four-hour drive. We arrived on Chincoteague just after one in the morning to find the tiny island fast asleep. We were staying at the Refuge Inn—or so we thought.

"We're all booked up, and I don't have any reservation in that last name!" the attendant informed us when we tried to check in.

"We mailed the check over a week ago," Rod said. "This is our honeymoon!"

"You gave our room away, didn't you?" I said. "We had to drive four hours!" I was tired, disappointed, angry, and about to cry.

Rod could tell how upset I was. "Then you'd better find us a room for the night."

"I'll see what I can do," the attendant said, not answering my question. He opened the phone book and made calls until he told us the Year of the Horse Inn, a bed and breakfast on the other side of the island, had a room. He said to return the next day, and he'd have a room for us.

The room at the Year of the Horse was okay, but it was no honeymoon suite. We didn't even have a bathroom to ourselves. We made the best of it though—it was our honeymoon, after all. When we returned to the Refuge the next day, the owner told us our deposit had just arrived, but I knew he was lying—just as the attendant had been lying the night before. Mail doesn't come on Sundays.

We stayed at The Refuge for the rest of our honeymoon, but any time we returned to the island after that, we refused to give them our business.

CHAPTER 14

I MAKE A CAREER

We settled into married life. We lived in the apartment in the basement of my parents' home in Shillington rent free for five years until we had saved enough to purchase our first home in Leesport. Our home in Leesport was several miles away from Rod's grandparents and his mom. I worked in a pre-school program with severely handicapped children at Easter Seals in Kenhorst, Pennsylvania, while Rod managed a local government program under the Comprehensive Employment and Training Act (CETA), which provided jobs training for public service workers. Jason lived with us every other weekend and took vacations with us as well.

We enjoyed our lives together. I was blessed to have a partner in my new husband, not a slave master. He respected me, and I respected him. I no longer lived in fear. *This is how marriage is supposed to be,* I thought gratefully, over and over again. And yet, something was missing, not in my marriage, but in my life. I was working for a paycheck at a job I liked but didn't love.

Rod must have noticed, because one day he asked me what I always wanted to do with my life—besides marry him, of course.

I had dreamed of becoming a cardiologist ever since we learned Dad had heart issues, but I knew that ship had sailed. I told him my second choice. "I always wanted to be a nurse," I said. "An RN."

"Then why don't you do that?" he said.

As if it's that easy, I said to myself, running through the thousands of reasons I couldn't do it: it was too late; I was too stupid; I had screwed up too much in high school and college; I had too many classes to make up; it would be too hard.

Then I had another idea. "What if I start as an LPN?" I said to Rod. "I could do that in a year at the vocational college. That way, I won't waste too much time and money if I can't hack it or don't like it." An RN is a registered nurse, and it takes two to four years to become an RN, depending upon if you choose an associate's degree versus a bachelor's degree program. Either way, you have the same responsibilities upon accepting a position. RNs typically do not provide direct patient care unless they work in a critical care setting. They are always in charge, make rounds with doctors, transcribe doctors' orders, and give out the medications. An LPN is a licensed practical nurse, a year-long program. LPNs provide direct patient care, except in a critical care setting, and they are guided by the RNs on duty.

Rod thought that would work. I called the next day and received an application, which I filled out and submitted. Much to my surprise, I was accepted for classes starting in August 1979, about four months after we were married. Eager to get started, I purchased all my books, uniforms, shoes, cap, and a lab coat.

I was nervous on the first day, but my teachers and fellow classmates were very gracious and helped me get back into the swing of things. I recognized Pam from Governor Mifflin and made friends with another student, named Joann from Shillington. By the end of the first week, we were commuting together.

I found medicine fascinating—this was the stuff of life. I wanted to learn more and more. When I really enjoyed a topic, I researched it in more detail outside of class for a greater understanding. I did excellent on the tests, too. I had a photographic memory—I could remember the most detailed information after I read over my notes several times, and I could recall all the details and charts by picturing them in my mind.

Sometimes Rod packed a picnic lunch, picked me up, and we drove a short distance to a local park. One day, I asked him why the sandwiches were so crunchy. I flipped over the top layer of bread and saw that he hadn't washed the mushrooms!

"You have to wash mushrooms?" he asked.

I almost threw up. "Really, Rod? Do you know what they grow mushrooms in? Manure. Horseshit. Haven't you ever smelled the Georgio Mushroom houses in Laureldale?"

"I'm sorry," he said sheepishly. He threw the rest of the sandwiches away. "I didn't know. Good thing I packed dessert." He made everything all right with his smile. But after that, I always checked any sandwich he made me. Trust but verify.

The first semester flew by. In the second semester, we started our clinical rotations through all the medical and surgical units at the Reading Medical Center, as well as a local nursing home and a mental hospital. We had to master all the nursing skills: bed making, listening to heart and breath sounds, assessing pulses and blood pressure, inserting a foley catheter, and so on. We learned to write care plans for our next day's assignments. These plans identified the patients' needs and ensured a collaboration among nurses, patients, and the other healthcare providers. Initially, we were in the hospital two days a week, with the other three days reserved for lectures. Eventually we were in the hospital four days a week.

The twelve months went by quickly and before I knew it, I was graduating. I surprised myself with how well I did, not only in clinical performance but also on tests and assignments. Upon graduation, I was presented with an award for clinical proficiency.

I loved medicine. Before I graduated, I had already applied and been accepted into an RN program at the local community college.

I passed my LPN boards with flying colors, and got a part-time job as an LPN on the cardiac-telemetry floor at the Reading Hospital.

Before I started my new job, Rod surprised me with a two-week vacation to California, so I could visit Shelley and Rod could meet her. I had never been to California, and I found the state beautiful, with its coastlines of jagged cliffs and beaches, its palm tree-lined streets, its attractive young people, its sprawling mission-style homes that all looked like mansions to me. Shelley took us to an art festival with juried artists, and I bought several pieces. We traveled to wine country and then all the way down the coastline into Mexico, where we spent some time in Ensenada at the famous dirt-floored Hussong's Cantina drinking local beer and too much tequila. While we were at the bar, Rod bought a bunch of Mexican blankets from the local peasants who wandered in and out of the bar. On our walk back to the hotel, Rod stepped off of the curb and lost his balance, going down on his knees. He wasn't hurt and didn't drop a blanket. We all laughed hysterically.

It was a good break after a year of school, and a good transition to my new career.

I found working with cardiac patients very rewarding. I could literally help them come back to life. Within a short time, the hospital had hired two cardiac and thoracic surgeons and established an open-heart unit. Our unit, E2 North, took the patients upon admission and also upon transfer from the open-heart behavioral intensive care unit (BICU). We admitted them the day before surgery for pre-op education, so they understood what was going to happen after surgery. We had them observe patients who had just come out of surgery—why they were on a ventilator, why they had to be in a medically induced coma, the need for bright lights and all of the activity around the patient.

A few weeks after I started working at the hospital, I also started working towards my RN, a decision I was very happy with. Though I enjoyed educating my patients about how diet, exercise, and better care of their heart would lengthen their lives, I wanted to do so much more than an LPN enabled me to do.

I continued as an LPN until I graduated with an associate's degree in the applied sciences and a minor in business administration. It took me three years of full-time commitment, but I graduated in the top ten percent of my nursing class. Upon graduation, I accepted a graduate nurse position at St. Joseph Hospital working in the intensive care unit (ICU) and coronary care unit (CCU). My nurse preceptor was Eileen, the Assistant Head Nurse. Every two weeks we rotated to the other unit.

By mid-summer I took and passed my RN boards with such a high score that I was eligible to work in any of the fifty states. Shortly after that, we took the three-month critical care course taught at the hospital by doctors and nurses. In these classes we learned at a deeper level and were trained how to apply it instantly in a clinical setting. We were now the eyes and ears of the critical care patients and their doctors. At the completion of every unit, we had to take exams to move on. I passed every one with flying colors.

I was excited to finally be able to take complete responsibility for the care of my patients without a preceptor. I also took on the charge nurse assignments. I oversaw the entire unit, giving and taking reports at the beginning and ending of the shift and rounding with the physicians. I had such a thirst for knowledge and wanted to provide the best of care to the sickest of patients in our inner-city hospital. I always requested to care for the most critically ill patients in the unit.

I thrived in this environment, perhaps because those who have survived trauma tend to seek jobs that provide an adrenalin rush. In critical care, I experienced that adrenalin rush every day. Whenever patients coded—had cardiac arrest due to their injuries or illnesses— we had to drop everything else to literally save their lives. We were hyperfocused and hyperaware, and the buzz of excitement would last for hours afterward.

I rotated from day shift to evenings or nights depending on the units' needs. When the two units were quiet, we were given the option to go home or cross-train in other specialties. I cross-trained with the dialysis unit, the medical detox unit, the intravenous team, and pediatrics. As critical care RNs, we often assisted in the emergency room, the recovery room, and the progressive care unit (PCU), the unit to which we typically sent our patients upon discharge from the critical care units.

I felt like I was doing exactly what I was supposed to be doing in my career—helping people, sometimes even saving their lives. Chalk up another one for Laura the fortune teller. I had become a healer.

Now that my career was taking off, though, things at home were going in the other direction. Rod was drinking more, and it was causing problems between us. Rod worked in the Commercial Department at Cartech, a specialty steel company, and a good part of his job was wining and dining customers. When customers were in town, Rod took them out to eat, then to drink, and often to strip clubs. He stayed out late and came home drunk, and if he didn't let me know ahead of time, I'd have dinner ready for us, and he wouldn't show up until after I had been long in bed—a replay of my father and mother's dynamic. We fought about all of this, but nothing changed. I thought we might be heading for divorce.

Then one evening, Rod was entertaining clients after work as he often did. After dinner they all went to a bar called R J Willoughby's for more drinks and to listen to music. After several more hours of drinking, they decided to drive to a strip club. Rod said he'd meet them there.

He never made it.

On his way to the bar in Wyomissing, he came up over a bridge too fast, lost control of his car, and took out several signs when his car struck the median. After his car came to a stop, he passed out at the wheel. He wasn't hurt, and neither was anyone else since it was a one-car accident. A Wyomissing police officer knocked on his window to wake him up. His car was towed, and he was taken to the Reading Hospital and Medical Center, where a blood alcohol test revealed he was twice the legal limit for Pennsylvania. He received a DUI citation.

I was at home in bed for the night when I got a call from the police officer. I was not happy, and not only because I had to get up, get dressed, and pick him up from the hospital. What was he thinking? What had he done to our family? I'm sure the ride home wasn't pleasant with me giving him an earful.

In the morning, he didn't dare ask me to take him to work, so he hitched a ride with a neighbor. Once there, he faced a Come-to-Jesus meeting with his superiors and human resources. They determined that if he wanted to remain an employee, he had to be treated at the Detox Unit at Reading Hospital. He called me at work (I was in the ICU that day) to let me know. I was shocked. I knew he drank a lot, but detox?

I visited him once while he was there. As crazy as this sounds, he had everyone, me included, convinced that he didn't have a problem with alcohol, that this was an isolated incident, and that he was only in detox to keep his job. He could sell ice to Alaskans! He even had the Cartech's Employee Assistance Program representative ready to sign off for his return to work.

Several hours before his discharge, however, a man in recovery came into the detox unit and declared, "Everyone who drinks is an alcoholic!" Rod took issue with that, and got up in the man's face, becoming belligerent and argumentative. That was a red flag to the counselors. Once they settled him down, they confronted him, and Rod finally admitted he did have a problem. The counselors notified the company, and Rod agreed to attend a thirty-day inpatient drug and alcohol treatment center—The Caron Foundation in Wernersville, Pennsylvania.

To visit him on Sundays, I had to attend a family education session, but I was still fairly skeptical about whether Rod needed treatment. Couldn't he just cut back on his own? But after my first visit, I changed my mind when I saw a different Rod. He apologized for all the times he stayed out drinking, and I didn't know where he was. He promised he would try harder to make our failing marriage work again! I was moved by this contrite, vulnerable Rod, especially when he told me how much he loved me and that he never wanted to lose me.

One of his counselors suggested I attend their five-day Family Program, which was also inpatient, so I could learn about living with an alcoholic and how it had affected me. I explained what was going on to my head nurse, Cathy, and she gave me the time off to attend the program. While there I was introduced to Al-Anon and educated about addiction and codependency. That's when I had a life-changing insight—I came from a long line of alcoholics and codependents, and I was both of these myself.

CHAPTER 15

ALCOHOLISM, PTSD, AND MY CODEPENDENT FAMILY

B y this time in my life—1985—I knew Dad was a drinker, and Mom couldn't control him. In fact, sometimes she joined him. I knew that when I was going through that awful year of sexual assault when I was thirteen, I drank until I blacked out so I wouldn't remember anything. I knew that since I was fifteen and could get into bars, my social life revolved around drinking, including my marriage to Rod. Now I won't exactly say that I thought all this was "normal"—whatever that means—but it was what it was. It's what we did. We didn't talk about it, much less put a name to it. It wasn't until the Caron family program that the lightbulb went off. Our family had a problem—more than one problem, really.

Bear with me while I put on my clinical hat.

Alcoholism is an emotionally, socially, and physically devastating disease affecting men and women of all ages and stages of life and all socioeconomic groups.[2] It's a family disease passed through our genes from one generation to the next. There is typically a pattern of heavy drinking that emerges despite the negative consequences. Those with a history of emotional or other kinds of trauma, as well as those with anxiety and depression, have an increased risk. In the alcoholic, unlike the non-alcoholic, there are changes that occur in the brain that make a person crave alcohol. Once they take a drink, they simply cannot have just one. They don't stop until they can no longer function. Some alcoholics drink daily, while others drink only on occasion, but all alcoholics have very little control of their drinking once they begin. Severe alcoholics often drink until they black out, and they suffer withdrawal symptoms—the DTs—when they go without.

In my own family, I realized that I, my father, mother, brother, nieces, nephews, aunts, and uncles all have alcoholic tendencies. In fact, one of my uncles died of end-stage alcoholism while in a hospital on a ventilator, a very sad and painfully slow death.

Alcohol was always served at family events, and it never seemed to run out. As a child, I hated when my parents drank too much because it usually ended in a fight. Even then, I was a people pleaser and peacemaker and felt I had to intervene, to fix it, to make it all better.

My father's alcoholism was compounded by PTSD from serving in two wars—WWII and Vietnam—as well as in cold war South Korea in the early sixties. He used alcohol to cope. At that time, PTSD wasn't talked about, and in fact very little was known about it. Soldiers simply didn't discuss their combat experiences when they returned home. It wasn't manly to do so.

I don't remember alcohol being a problem until Dad returned from Korea. He drank more in the house in the evenings and on weekends, and when he went out to drink he missed dinners and didn't come home till the early hours of the morning.

After his return from Vietnam, his drinking grew even more out of control.

Dad's assignment after Vietnam was Fort Dix, New Jersey, where he was promoted to Chief Warrant Officer 2. Many nights he didn't come home from work, but stopped at the Officer's Club, where he drank for hours. At some point, he'd call Mom to let her know where he was. She'd already be angry because she had made dinner for all of us, and we had eaten hours before. Eventually he'd stumble into the house, and that was when the fights began. Instead of eating the dinner she was now trying to reheat, Dad headed straight to the refrigerator for another beer. More than once, he stumbled, and the bottle slipped out of his hand and shattered on the kitchen floor, beer and brown glass flying everywhere. "Don't come in here," she called to me and Kevin. "I don't want anyone to get cut." Then she yelled at Dad, "Get the hell out of here. You've made such a mess in here and you certainly don't need another damn beer. Go to bed!"

I'd feel sick to my stomach. It always worried me when he came home like this. The screaming fights upset me. I was terrified they'd get a divorce, and our family would break up. My brother just went to bed and fell asleep. That was his way of coping. I lay awake for what seemed like an eternity, willing them to stop fighting.

Other times I retreated to my room but could hear the screaming over the loud music I played as a distraction. Finally, in desperation, I left my room, crying, "Please, please stop fighting! I can't stand to hear you guys screaming at each other anymore!" I became the Little Mother in the house, the peacemaker, because usually by then they'd both be drunk. I screamed so loud my throat hurt. The next day it sounded like I had laryngitis.

After Dad was discharged from the army about a year later, he was devastated. He became very depressed. He was only forty-four years old and forced to live life as a "cardiac cripple," as he described it. Dad had owned a plumbing business before he had re-enlisted in the Army, but he wasn't a plumber anymore. He wasn't sure how he could support his family outside the military. He was career Army, that was his identity, and he looked every bit the part, with his flat-top haircut, his tall frame, chiseled by years of intense physical work, his command presence. Heads turned when he entered a room. He shouted commands whenever he needed something. When that was all taken from him, as he saw it, he was nothing anymore, and there was nothing to keep the PTSD at bay. He drank to fill the vacuum, and this supercharged the PTSD. His behavior became a little crazy.

In the late sixties, practically overnight, Dad became paranoid about the civil rights protests. Crazy paranoid. My brother and I had finished our chores and were headed to the local swimming pool one day. It was just after lunch when he summoned us to our kitchen. "Sit down," he said, his jittery eyes indicating he had already been drinking heavily, the odor of cigarettes and beer coming off him in waves. Speaking slowly but loudly, Dad warned us, "The negroes are coming to Shillington with guns to take hostages. If you see a crowd of negroes at the pool, run home as fast as you can! Understand?"

"Yes," we both responded, knowing enough not to argue.

What Dad told us scared me, but later Kevin reassured me. "Don't worry. That's never going to happen here." We swam most of the afternoon and came home just before dinner, walking in on a bit of a situation.

After we had left for the pool, Dad continued drinking, and grew more agitated and more convinced we were about to be invaded. In defense, he gathered all the sharp knives in the house and hid them in the kitchen freezer. Mom was trying to reason with him when we arrived. "That makes no damn sense," she said. "They're not going to break into the house and kill us with our own knives!" She moved toward the refrigerator, but he blocked her way. "Let me put the knives back!"

I could see the anger in Mom's face as she fought a losing battle against Dad's paranoid fantasies. I couldn't take it any longer. I tried to get them to stop in my normal voice, then I raised it a little louder, but they kept at it, and finally I screamed, "PLEASE STOP! I'm begging you!" as loud as I could. Mom stopped her end of it, came to my side, held me in her arms. "It's okay, Kim. We'll stop."

And they would stop for a while, but then they'd always start up again. "Why do you always have to drink so much?" Mom would demand of my father. Mom was never short on words and delivered them quite eloquently for a farm girl forced to quit school after eighth grade to help support their large family during the Great Depression.

Dad was used to giving orders rather than taking them. "I think I'm old enough to decide what and when I'll drink!" he'd yell back, smelling of Old Spice and beer.

Mom would mumble something and leave whatever room they were fighting in.

The military doctors prescribed sedatives, sleeping pills, and anti-depressants. Most days Dad washed the pills down with beer. After a while, Dad got tired of lugging so many cases of beer home from the distributor. He took all the shelves out of the kitchen refrigerator and installed a keg instead. Problem solved. Mom had to put most of our food in a second refrigerator in the basement since only a few things could fit around the keg.

Dad was a man of few words, but he opened up when drinking, and I learned to take advantage of that. That's how I learned everything I know about his war experiences in Italy, Korea, and Vietnam, as well as his family and childhood, stories I passed on to my own children. They always marvel at how many times their grandfather cheated death, and are very proud of him. He may have left behind a legacy of damage, but there was also a lot of love there. He was a complicated man, my father.

Despite all that, Dad lived into his nineties. Except for a couple of months in 2010 when he lived with us and Mom in Arizona before my mother's death in 2011, he managed to live in his own home despite being legally blind until his death on July 14, 2016, at 92 years of age. He was about to sell his home and move to Arizona to live with us, but he had a massive heart attack and died in Reading Hospital.

In the end, I had become very close to Dad, and losing him was difficult. It was only later in life that he could he tell me openly that he loved me, and I cherished that time with him. His funeral at Arlington National Cemetery was spectacular, almost presidential, at least to me. He was taken to his grave by a horse-drawn caisson with full military honors. After the ceremony, a lone bugler played Taps, which was followed by a 21-gun salute. As they marched out of the cemetery, the military band played, "When the Saints Go Marching In." It was a beautiful and moving tribute for a man who had given so much to the Army and the country he loved.

+ + +

Like my father, my mother had had her own wars to fight, though they weren't of the military kind, and also experienced PTSD.

Farm life during the Great Depression was difficult. The family farm could sustain them with beef, chicken, pork, eggs, vegetables, and fruits, but they still needed money for other essentials. The oldest two girls were required to quit school after eighth grade to earn money for their family. For the seven boys it was mandatory to complete high school and then obtain a job or enlist in the military.

My mom's first job was to take care of her cousin and best friend, Eleanor. Eleanor lived next to their farm, so Mom walked there daily through the meadow and across the stream. Eleanor had a severe congenital heart defect known as Tetralogy of Fallot. This presents as four separate defects within the heart. Today surgery can correct the defects, but in the 1930s there was no treatment.

As a child, Eleanor was too sick to play outside. Mom prepared and ate breakfast with her before allowing her to rest. She tired easily due to her constant struggle to breathe. Eleanor's lips, fingers, and feet were always blue in color and her breathing was rapid and labored. Her legs were three times normal size and a pale-yellow fluid wept like tears from her pores. Her fingertips and the tips of her toes were oddly shaped. She could scarcely walk due to the fluid retention and shortness of breath. She was a prisoner to her chair, propped upright with pillows.

Mom brought the outside world to Eleanor, and Eleanor loved her for this. When it snowed, she'd carry snow inside in a large pail and let

Eleanor feel it and mold it into figures before it melted. In the summer, Mom would pick cattails and flowers from the meadow and arrange them in a container within Eleanor's reach. Mom and Eleanor were inseparable. Some nights Mom stayed long after both of her parents had gotten home from work. When Mom did go home, Eleanor longed to go along with her. She often cried for Mom, especially when she had bouts of breathing difficulty. As time passed, Eleanor's condition worsened, making it much more difficult to play and laugh with Mom. Mom read adventure books to her, or they sat quietly and drew pictures together.

One day, suddenly, Eleanor became extremely short of breath. As Mom desperately tried to comfort her, she noticed that Eleanor's entire body was turning a deep blue. Not wanting to leave her alone to go for help, Mom sat beside her and gently held her in her arms while reminding her that her struggle would soon pass, and she would be okay. Mom gently stroked Eleanor's hair to move it away from her face and gently rubbed her arms and face, telling her how much she loved her. As Mom gave her a hug, Eleanor took her last earthly breath. My mother's best friend was suddenly gone forever. No one that she had ever loved this deeply had ever left her. She felt lost, alone, and empty—and guilty. Was it her fault? Should she have gone for help? She mourned Eleanor's death for many years.

Sometime after Mom's death, I found a Christmas card from Eleanor telling Mom how much she loved her. The card was in perfect condition, not tattered by the seventy-five or more years Mom had saved it. Today that card hangs in my living room, matted and framed. It would have made her so happy to see the beautiful picture and its final resting place.

As a child, I recall Mom talking about Eleanor many times, but she always omitted the one important detail—that she had died in Mom's arms. Mom finally told me the rest of the story before she passed away. That's when I realized that just like my dad and me, Mom had dealt with PTSD silently because no one knew what it was in the 1930s.

Unlike my father and me, she did not resort to alcohol as a coping mechanism. She became codependent instead.

Even before Eleanor's death, growing up in a large family, where everyone had to contribute and help with the care of younger siblings, Mom was set up for codependency early in life. One of her younger sisters thought my mom was her mom. She was very upset when Mom got married, thinking Mom had abandoned her.

This all led to Mom's very dysfunctional, codependent relationship with Dad. This dysfunctionality increased tenfold after his first heart attack. Mom did everything she could to make Dad happy and to make life easier for him. She prepared heart healthy meals. She tried to keep the house quiet. She listened to his diatribes. She tried to soothe him.

Dad, on the other hand, always did whatever he wanted, and Mom not only permitted it, she enabled it. This form of learned behavior—codependency—is typically passed down from one generation to another. It is not surprising that I would become a nurse or my children would follow suit as a teacher and a doctor, always in the role of caring for others. Codependency also affects one's ability to have healthy relationships. Codependent people usually form or maintain relationships that are one-sided, emotionally destructive, and sometimes abusive. It is not surprising then that I ended up in an abusive first marriage and that my life has been affected by alcohol.

The partners of codependents are typically chemically dependent or suffer from a chronic or mental illness. My dad had all three: he was an alcoholic; he had heart disease; and he suffered PTSD and depression. The codependent partner will always do more than their share, all the time. Mom's older sister was very lazy and never did her fair share. When asked to assist with a chore, she headed to the outhouse. Mom caught her many times sitting in the outhouse pretending the Sears Catalog was a church hymnal as she sang some of her favorite songs.

The result was that Mom must have lost touch with her own wants and needs at a very early age. Mom always supported the underdog and always defended those in need and those she loved. Mom felt like she had to take care of everyone all the time, even strangers. If she saw a mother with kids juggling too much in a store, she'd stop and help them.

One person Mom helped was Gwen, a woman who lived in our town. I was friends with her daughter Jane, and my brother Kevin had dated her daughter Ann. Gwen had schizophrenia. She walked around town with her long blonde hair and bright red lipstick, stopped suddenly, and started yelling to no one, her arms flailing. Gwen enjoyed her beer, and stopped at Johnny's Cafe or at the bar of the restaurant where my mom worked as a waitress—Ibach's Seafood. Gwen had become a laughingstock, and Mom thought that wasn't right—that she was still a human being deserving compassion.

After Mom finished work, she'd go into the bar and ask Gwen if she wanted to come home with her for a visit. Gwen loved Mom, who brought her home many times. Gwen would have some beers, eat some snacks, and when Mom got too tired, she would drive Gwen home. No one else in our town ever invited Gwen over.

Mom certainly did not drink to the extent and frequency my father did, but she had her own issues with alcohol. I saw her drunk on many occasions. But where Dad was an ornery drunk, Mom was a silly drunk and more pleasant to be around. Perhaps I'm underplaying it, though. Like me, she experienced blackouts when she drank too much. I remember her saying she didn't remember parts of some drunken nights.

One night my girlfriend Val and I went out with my parents to the local American Legion. We had fun, playing music on the jukebox, dancing, and, of course, drinking. Val and I were talking and laughing with Mom most of the evening, and at some point we had to hit the ladies room. An ugly, dusty vase of deep orange, harvest gold, and olive-green plastic flowers sat on the counter in front of the mirror. "Look at these ugly things," Mom said, then plucked the leaves and flowers one by one and tossed them in the air. We laughed while we grabbed her hand like she was a naughty child and led her back to our table.

When Mom wasn't drinking or fighting with Dad, she was the kindest, most generous, honest Christian I've ever met. But even her fights with Dad were an attempt to take care of him. She taught us at a very young age to pray before each meal and at bedtime while we knelt beside our bed. She kept her Bible beside her bed, where I saw her sitting to read it. She made sure we attended Sunday School, got baptized, got confirmed, and joined and attended a church that felt like home. She did everything for us—for her family, and very much to her loss. But she never would have seen it that way. That's how she showed us her love.

I suppose that not everyone has a close relationship with their mother, but in my case, I always had a good one. As a small child, my mom was someone I loved unconditionally, and I knew she loved me unconditionally as well. She was always kind and compassionate and slow to anger. Even when she was angry, she never lost her cool. She laughed often but never at others. She liked to play games. She always rooted for the underdog, helped those in need, and taught her children to do the same. She was a hard worker both at home and at work. She was busy from sunrise until long after dark every day, including weekends. She prepared and served three meals each day and baked homemade desserts from scratch. She even baked homemade bread, just like her mom. She instilled the good habits in her children. She always told me it was important to make the world a better place for the next generation.

We knew and loved each other on the deepest level a mother and daughter can reach. While I was going through some of the breast surgeries I'll write about later in the book, Mom had advanced dementia. After one surgery, Dad told me that for the previous two days, my mother had been in great pain. He had given her pain medicine, but she kept saying that she wished her Kimmie could be with her.

The mother-daughter connection in reverse, I thought. As a child, whenever I didn't feel well, all I wanted was the company of my mother. I cried for a long time after we hung up the phone. Because I couldn't travel, all I could do was pray for her. The love between a mother and daughter is such a special, genuine, and deeply committed connection. Mom always knew I loved her, and I reminded her again and again of how special she was. I was so blessed that she always knew who her family was until the day she passed through those "Pearly Gates." I had talked to her almost every day of my life. For the last three months of her life, she lived with us in Arizona.

My mother passed away on January 25, 2011, at the age of 86. I was heartbroken. I did her eulogy at her Celebration of Life at the brownstone church in Pennsylvania she had attended all her life. Her grandfather had helped build that church with stones from their farm. I also did a eulogy at her funeral at Arlington National Cemetery, where she was buried on March 8, 2011. (My father was eligible to be buried at Arlington because of his rank, and once he signed on, Mom was also eligible as his spouse.) In both eulogies, I said much of what I've written here—about her strong Christian faith, her unconditional love for her family and everyone else in the world, her quiet strength.

I longed to have children of my own so I could instill the same characteristics in them. When Adam and Sarah were born, I had my grandmother's and mother's examples to draw on. It is no wonder that I have great relationships with my grown children. As Adam said, we now know one another on a different level since my accident.

My relationship with Sarah is akin to what I had with my mom. We have been much more than a mother and daughter. As Sarah got older, we'd shop together, and she always gave me her honest opinion, solicited or unsolicited, about how something fit or what it looked like. It was like I gave birth to my biggest critic and my best friend. We've had hours of pants-splitting laughter, but we've shed many tears as well. Friend, foe, mother, daughter, and so much more. Sarah has never been, nor will ever be, a people pleaser like her mama. That is a blessing I am grateful for, and I'd like to think I had something to do with that, with teaching her a better way, with breaking the cycle of people pleasing and codependency. Something Mom would be proud of—passing on strength to the next generation.

....

CHAPTER 16

WE GO TO REHAB

C aron's family program was eye-opening. I gained insight into much of my family's dysfunction. I identified myself as the people pleaser in my own addicted family, the one who constantly gave of myself to make everyone else happy. I also filled the role of the lost child in my dysfunctional family's dynamics, the child who becomes invisible, who retreats from conflict by spending a lot of time alone or out of the house, who immerses herself in outside activities so she doesn't have to feel what she's feeling.

This described me to the T.

I had retreated from my family, staying under the radar by hiding in my bedroom or the basement when I was home and by spending as much time out of the house as possible, at parties, at activities, at the houses of friends who I thought had a more normal family life. I learned other things about the lost child in the program. The lost child never reveals the family's skeletons in the closet. They hide the shame—their own and their family's—from everyone. The lost child learns that their needs don't matter. The lost child both wants desperately to be heard, but is terrified of being heard lest they don't measure up to expectations. The psychologist Donald Winnicott puts it this way: for a child, "It is a joy to be hidden, but disaster not to be found."[3]

We watched a movie about addiction and I had an AHA moment: I was an alcoholic myself—it wasn't just the people around me. It was a great awakening, but tough to swallow. When it was my turn to talk after the movie, I let everyone know I was an alcoholic in need of treatment—a codependent alcoholic, to be exact.

For that reason, before the family program ended, I decided that I, too, should attend a thirty-day inpatient program. Since the Caron Foundation had more than one site, I wouldn't have to attend the same one as Rod. Cathy, my Head Nurse, gave me the thirty days off and agreed to keep everything confidential.

Rod's accident ended up being the blessing we both needed to become whole, though Rod was surprised when I told him I was going into rehab, as was my family. They all thought it was Rod who had the problem and needed rehab. Of course, *his* family thought it was only *me* who had the problem and needed rehab (conveniently forgetting that very small matter of Rod's accident and DUI). I laugh about it now. That's one of the things I learned in rehab and therapy—the mental gymnastics individuals and families go through to claim that nothing is wrong with *them*. It's always somebody else who has the problem, whatever it may be.

My drinking was always tied to the rapes and the PTSD that resulted.

Considering how I hated what alcohol had done to my family as a kid, it is ironic, but not surprising, that I would resort to alcohol to cope. I suppose I turned to alcohol because it was readily available and because I had the alcoholic genes. I also had to deal with the effects of PTSD—the nightmares, the paranoia, the shame and guilt, the screaming voices in my head—on my own, since I hadn't reported the crime. Now I know that it would have made a lot more sense to tell my parents what had happened on that first night. I could have saved myself from the months of torture that followed, and they could have gotten me the help I desperately needed.

Being raped affected all aspects of my life. I lost faith in myself. I thought I was a bad person, that I had done something to bring this on. Was it the way I dressed or something I said? I stopped doing well in school because I didn't feel as if I deserved to do well in school. I didn't feel I deserved much of anything. I hung out in bars as soon as I could pass for legal because at least there I felt as if I belonged. It has taken me a rehab program and years of therapy to get past these feelings, and honestly, I'm not always sure I have completely gotten past them.

Despite what our families thought, we both accepted we were alcoholics and needed to work the twelve-step program that Alcoholics Anonymous prescribed. My parents visited me on Sundays during my time at Caron. According to my treatment plan, I needed to level with them so they could understand why I had begun drinking so young. At this point, Rod and my treatment group were the only ones who knew I had been raped. When I told my parents, Dad just kind of shut down, but Mom wanted to know who it was.

"Who was it, Kim? Tell me who it was. I've got a thing or two to say to him. This is terrible. Unthinkable. Why didn't you tell us?"

"I was afraid, Mom. I was afraid to tell anyone. He threatened me. He threatened all of you! I thought I could get through it myself."

"Tell me now. It's not too late.

"I can't. I'm not sure why. I just can't."

"Why are you protecting him? Please, just tell me his name."

"I told Rod what happened after we were married, but I didn't tell him his name either."

"Give me his name! He deserves an ass kicking. Dad will kick his ass. *I* will kick his ass! Just give me a name."

This was another thing I learned in rehab and therapy. That loved ones feel so helpless in the face of such information that they get angry and strike out at something they think they can control.

"No, I'm sorry. I can't tell you. We better get in line for lunch before we miss it." I stood up and gestured toward the line. I was relieved that

I had told her, but I did wonder why I didn't want to give his name—out of strength or weakness, I couldn't tell.

Once Rod completed his thirty days, he visited me when he could. My experience at Caron was positive. It was the safe place I needed to begin healing. I loved the people in my group—we were all on the same journey for different reasons. I made friends with a woman named Joy. Though we weren't in the same small group, Joy and I sat together during our large group meetings and at meals. During free time, we walked the grounds for exercise. She was a single mom and had one son who was less than ten at the time. I finished my thirty days before Joy, and we exchanged addresses and phone numbers. Initially, we kept in fairly close contact, but over the years, we communicated less and less. We still send Christmas cards encouraging each other to stay sober.

As the result of intense group therapy as well as one-to-one counseling, I learned about myself, addiction, and codependency. I also knew there was so much more to learn that as my discharge day approached, I wasn't sure I was ready to leave. I knew that I felt safer in that environment than I had in a long time, and I didn't want to drink again. I wasn't sure I could stand fast on the outside, a natural and normal reaction, I was told, an important step I had to take. I wouldn't be entirely on my own, though. Since I was a local resident, my aftercare counseling would also be conducted at Caron. And I planned to go to ninety AA meetings in ninety days, as recommended by the program to help with the transition.

After breakfast on the morning I was going home, I rang the bell that signified I had completed my thirty days, then said my goodbyes to everyone just before Rod arrived to pick me up. Rod was happy he was going to have me home again. The program had been an unexpected healing for both of us, but my discharge was bittersweet. I was the only one leaving that day, and I'd be returning to work the very next day filled with trepidation about this new me facing the world sober.

This was in 1985. I am proud to say that I haven't touched alcohol since. Entering that program was one of the best things I have ever done.

My head nurse had visited me during my stay at Caron. I asked her if she could plan a mandatory staff meeting for the morning I returned to work. I wanted to tell everyone where I had been, and why. She agreed to arrange the meeting.

The following morning, I left the house early and bought six dozen donuts. Everyone welcomed me with open arms and thanked me for my honesty and courage. Later that day, I asked the head nurse if I could teach the new critical care class on alcoholism and addiction. So many of the young critical care nurses I worked with also used alcohol to suppress the horrors they faced daily taking care of critically ill patients. If I could pass on what I had learned about myself, maybe I could help a few of my colleagues. She agreed, so that evening I got to work on the lecture. Several nurses I worked with went into treatment after I had paved the way.

Being sober wasn't all sunshine and roses though. Without the layers of protection afforded by alcohol, I faced the world naked and alone and began doubting myself. I questioned my competence. As a critical care nurse with years of experience, I had never made a mistake that jeopardized the health or well-being of my patients, but now that I was sober, I felt like an imposter. What right did I have to make these life and death decisions? Soon everyone would realize that I didn't know anything. I'd be exposed and hounded out of the profession in shame and humiliation.

I didn't know why I felt this way. Intellectually, I knew I was a damn good nurse, but I *felt* this overwhelming fear that I was going to fall on my face, that I was walking on eggshells, and it would only be a matter of time before I was outed as the ultimate imposter. In response, I drove myself harder and harder at work, raking myself over the coals for the most minor inconsistencies I wouldn't think of mentioning if another nurse had done the same thing. I became my own worst critic.

I did some research and found that Imposter Syndrome is an actual condition, one that affects women more than men. The women affected are typically highly intelligent and high achieving, but find it difficult to accept that their accomplishments are the result of their own competence rather than good fortune. That was me! When others praised my talents, I wrote off my successes to timing and good luck. I felt inadequate! My self-esteem crumbled, and self-doubt plagued me for the rest of the years I worked in critical care.

Then one day, as I was thinking about some of the things I learned in rehab and AA's twelve steps, it hit me. I was so busy forgiving everyone else that I had never gotten around to forgiving myself. I wasn't an imposter. I was riddled with unforgiveness, and it was eating me alive. I beat myself up for every single misstep of my life, whether real or perceived. No wonder I felt as I did.

It was one of the toughest things I've ever done, but also one of the best. When I let go and forgave myself for the things that were out of my control, the healing that had begun in rehab deepened, and I embraced this new person I had become.

To stay sober and avoid the temptations that lead to relapse, Rod and I both changed people, places, and things as recommended by AA—we didn't hang out with people who centered their lives on drinking, and we certainly stayed away from bars. Further, we both started to tell our stories at AA speaker meetings to commit more fully to sobriety, and we spoke at local high schools to educate kids about addiction. It wasn't easy, but we were committed.

To take some of the pressure off, I left critical care to take a nurse consultant position at Aetna Insurance. I loved my new role. I worked the day shift, with no weekends, no holidays, and no crazy last-minute calls to work so-and-so's shift at midnight. It was a revelation. Was this how most people lived and worked?

Soon I had another reason to be grateful for the job change. At twenty-nine years old, after what seemed like an eternity, I was pregnant with our first child.

CHAPTER 17

OUR FAMILY GROWS: A BOY AND A GIRL

The morning sickness hit immediately, the first sign I was pregnant. *Why do they call it morning sickness when it lasts all day?* I thought every time I threw up. Which was all the time. When I brushed my teeth. When I took a shower. When I ate too much, or didn't eat enough. Sometimes for no reason at all. I was embarrassed when it happened in public, even though I kept saltines and hard candies in my purse. Small, frequent meals seemed to help. Over the course of the next few months, I was even able to put on a few pounds, as the doctor requested, despite the vomiting.

Work was going great, and I was grateful I was no longer in critical care. Odd shifts, weekends, and holidays would have been so much harder. In the ICU, I also would have been exposed to infections and contagious illnesses, including HIV. *I'm very lucky*, I thought to myself.

The ultrasound suggested a girl, though not definitively. We had narrowed down the girl's name to Ashley, but we weren't sure about a boy's name. Rod wanted a Rod junior, but I pulled rank and told him there was no way I was naming our son Rodney. Maybe as a middle name. Nor did I particularly want a junior who would always be compared to his daddy.

It was almost two weeks until I was due—January 11. I was scheduled to see the doctor twice a week in these last stages. I had decided on an epidural for pain control, and for labor I had picked out some soothing, tranquil music that included sounds of the beach.

On December 30, 1986, I woke up to a very sick husband. Rod had a high fever and body aches. Since food was out of the question, I tried to get him to drink more fluids so he wouldn't dehydrate.

"Whatever you do, don't have the baby today. I'm too sick!" Rod sniffled.

"That's sort of out of my control, but I'll say a prayer for you," I said.

He went back to sleep.

I still had one more load of baby items to wash and put away and grocery shopping to complete. At two in the afternoon, I sat down to eat lunch—a coconut, buttercream cake with strawberries on top. When I bent over to put my plate in the dishwasher, I felt a twinge in my back, like menstrual cramps, but I never had them there before. Maybe I just needed to go to the bathroom. I sat down, and felt a rush of fluid. My water had broken! I was in labor! So much for not having the baby that day.

"Rod, are you awake?" I hollered.

"Yes, what is it?" he said in a raspy voice.

"I'm pretty sure my water broke," I said.

Within five seconds, he was at the bathroom door, holding onto the wicker dresser. "I feel like I'm going to pass out," he said. "You weren't supposed to have the baby for two more weeks!"

"Babies come when babies come."

"I have to go back to bed. I feel awful." He went into the bedroom.

"I'm calling the doctor. Maybe Kelly can take me to the hospital."

The nurse told me to go directly to the hospital. Next, I called Kelly at Aetna, and she said she'd be right there. The cramps were still irregular, so I took a quick shower, pausing whenever the pain got too intense.

When Kelly arrived, she said, "How are you doing?"

"My contractions are getting more intense." I gripped my abdomen.

"Let's go then."

I called Mom, said goodbye to Rod, then grabbed the bag I had packed weeks ago. Kelly normally drove more slowly than I did, but that day she didn't waste any time. My contractions were getting more intense and more frequent, so when Kelly spotted a police officer about a mile from the hospital, she flagged him down to request a police escort. All he did was shake his head and point to the hospital.

"Thanks for nothing," Kelly snapped. She turned into the emergency room drop-off and jogged to the vestibule to get me a wheelchair.

I waited for a contraction to pass, then swung into the wheelchair. Kelly pushed me into the intake area and announced, "She's in labor!"

A nice young girl took over the wheelchair and pushed me towards the elevator. "I'll take you upstairs," she said.

My contractions were getting stronger and more frequent. Once upstairs, Kelly helped me change. A nurse inserted an intravenous line and my doctor examined me. I was only two centimeters dilated. I thought I'd be further along as bad as the contractions had been. This was the worst pain I had ever had. I had a new appreciation for what my mom went through with the three of us. I put on the headphones playing the sound of the sea.

By early evening, Rod arrived along with my parents. When Dr. Kleiner saw how sick he was, he asked him to put a mask on whenever he came into the room. He also thought Rod might be better off sleeping in the waiting room while Kelly helped me with labor.

I had the electrodes from a TENS unit attached to my abdominal muscles to relax them with electrical impulses. I also had an epidural for pain relief, but I had a "hot spot," a small area where the nerve block didn't take. I could still feel the contractions. Meanwhile, the sounds of the ocean weren't doing anything for me. I yanked the headphones out of my ears and tossed them across the room with a few choice words! Next, I ripped the TENS unit off my stomach and tossed that across the room as well. The contractions were just too intense at this point. Kelly laughed every time I threw something.

Labor wasn't progressing. A resident examined me and discovered that the baby was in a posterior position. They had to manually turn the baby in the opposite direction, so he could continue down the birth canal headfirst. When I saw the doctor's arms inside me up to his elbows, I thanked the Lord for the epidural!

They also placed a fetal head monitor onto the scalp of the baby to monitor distress. At one point Rod came back into the room, fully masked, and announced that he was feeling better. He had slept and then gone downstairs to eat an egg salad sandwich from a vending machine. At his description of the sandwich, I projectile vomited across the room. Kelly moved fast to clean it, and Rod shut up.

The next time the doctor examined me, I was ten centimeters dilated. They unlocked my bed and wheeled me toward the delivery room. Rod and Kelly were given OR caps to enter the delivery room. By ten at night, I started feeling all the urges to push, but the nurse kept telling me, "Hold off! Don't push until you get into the delivery room."

By 10:29 our first child was born. We named him Adam Michael. Upon birth and within five minutes, his APGAR scores were all normal, which meant he was healthy. I offered a prayer of thanks.

We actually had some trouble naming our son. We were told we were having a girl early on, so we didn't have any boys' names ready. I had already told Rod I wasn't naming my kid Rodney, so Rodney, Junior, was out of the question. Michael is Rod's and Jason's middle name, so that was easy. On the morning of our discharge, I had come up with Joshua or Daniel. I asked Rod if he had a preference, and we decided on Joshua Michael. When I got off of the phone, I told my roommate the name. "That's our dog's name!" she said.

Oh, no, I thought and called Rod back and told him about the dog. I flipped through our name book, and one name popped off the page. "Adam!" I said.

"Adam it is," Rod agreed.

I was in the hospital for New Year's Eve and went home on New Year's Day, which had received a fresh white blanket of snow and ice.

Adam looked tiny, like a small peanut, in his enormous car seat. Over the first week, his bilirubin level had risen to a rather high level, so we had to dress him in a diaper only and expose him to sunlight to bring his levels down. We called him Billy Rubin.

Once the bilirubin leveled off, Adam developed colic and was constantly in pain. We tried everything to soothe the poor boy. His pain got worse, which took a toll on me as well. Sometimes I'd watch him while he slept, and I could tell from the way his stomach contorted that he was in pain, long before he'd wake up screaming. Thank God for my mom, who came to our house almost daily. On his worst days, Adam cried twenty out of twenty-four hours. Sometimes I'd rock him and cry along. Was this what it meant to be a mother? Since he wasn't gaining weight, either his pediatrician had me supplement the breast feedings with a special formula. His doctor tried to encourage me by saying that by three months all this would pass, but I wasn't buying it. Each day was an eternity; anything more than that was unimaginable!

Then, just as his doctor had predicted, one day Adam had colic and the next day, he didn't, and it never returned again. He began thriving then, gaining weight, and growing.

Once the colic passed—about three months after we brought him home—I went back to work part-time in the ICU and CCU at St. Joseph's. We settled into a new rhythm—feeding, diapering, working, playing—and life went on.

Adam was twenty months old when I started throwing up again and knew I was pregnant with our second child. We had recently moved into a new home, with much more space. I hoped to have a girl this time.

I had accepted a new position in critical care at Pottstown Hospital, where I worked two twelve-hour night shifts every week-end and was compensated as a full-time RN. The problem was, I had a forty-minute drive home after a twelve-hour shift, and once I was pregnant, I regularly nodded off while driving. The wheel would jerk me awake with my heart racing. I'd pull off of the road and take a nap, even though I knew Rod would be worried. After the toughest nights, I sometimes fell asleep more than once. Most mornings, I'd blast music and roll down the windows to keep me awake. When it got warmer that spring of 1989, I'd blast the air conditioner. Rod would get so upset when I finally arrived home, but what else could I do? I had to work.

Everyone guessed I was going to have another boy, but Mom and I both thought it was a girl. At one of my appointments, the doctor asked rather snidely, "Have you decided what medication you plan to use this time. You didn't particularly care for the pain last time!"

I was speechless. *Let's see you shit out a football, then we'll discuss it, you snide son of a bitch*, I thought. But what I said was, "I plan on an epidural." I also planned to get a female ob-gyn after this baby was born.

It was mid-April, with just over two weeks left until my due date. I was really uncomfortable. Sleep was nearly impossible, and because the baby had dropped into my lower abdomen, I always felt like I had a full bladder. I planned to work the next two weekends before mater-nity leave.

One Saturday evening I was the charge nurse in coronary care. The charge nurse generally assigned fewer patients to herself so she had time for the other duties overseeing the unit. That night, I had one patient while the other nurses had two. So, when the nursing supervisor called at about three in the morning to send over an over-flow patient who was recovering from anesthesia after a C-section, I assigned her to me. The problem was, the patient had shot heroin just before she came to the hospital, and lost the baby to fetal distress.

"Kim, you can't do that," Nancy said after I filled her in. "It'll be too tough. I'll take her."

"Nope, I can't do that to you," I said. "She's my patient."

Once the patient was set up in Room 1, I monitored her as I would monitor any other. Whenever I was inside her room, though, I couldn't help but tear up. All I could think was how badly I wanted a little girl. And this mother had cared more about heroin than keeping her poor little girl healthy. When I left the room, I cried so hard each time my coworkers hugged me. I understood addiction. I'd been through recovery and had taught others about it as well. But I struggled to feel compassion toward this woman.

When she came to, she asked me, "Can you get my baby for me so I can hold her?"

I must have looked at her in horror, because then she said, "I know she's gone. I just want to see her."

"I'll call my supervisor," I said.

Someone would have to remove the body from the body bag and wrap it in a blanket. In a few minutes, the automatic doors opened to a nun carrying the swaddled baby, which she handed to me in a white blanket. I silently prayed, *Lord, help me get through this!*

I handed her to the mother, and, following my supervisor's instructions, stayed in the room.

My emotions were all over the place. The mother in me wanted to call the police, but the nurse in me knew I had to protect my patient's rights and confidentiality. Still, I kept thinking, "It's not fair. She caused the death of her baby." Then in the next second, I pitied her addiction. *There but for the grace of God ....* Before I got sober, how many times had I driven after a few too many?

She moved the blanket to see the baby's face, and both of us cried, tears pouring down our cheeks. Then she said, "I want to see if she has ten fingers and toes." She unwrapped the swaddled infant.

It's a little late for that, I thought. All that I hoped and dreamed about was having a girl, and this woman had thrown it away.

I was relieved when she finally kissed her baby, then re-wrapped her and handed her to me. When I left the room, I called my nursing supervisor to come to the unit and get the adorable, dead infant. She sensed my distress and immediately came through the double doors to return the baby to the morgue. Much later, I wondered where the nun had come from, Pottstown Hospital was not a Catholic hospital, but in my own distress, I never asked.

That morning I didn't fall asleep on the way home because I cried most of the drive. When I got home and told Rod what had happened, he was upset I had to deal with that.

"It's time to start your maternity leave, now. You're done. You're not going back next weekend. Call your head nurse."

"You're right. I'm exhausted. A dead baby with two weeks to go! It's too much. It's just too much."

I grabbed a yogurt from the refrigerator, and sat down next to Adam, who was eating breakfast in his usual messy way, with cereal on the floor and mashed into his hair. He looked at me with his bright, trusting eyes. How could any mother ...? No, I didn't even want to think about it.

I had an appointment with my OB/GYN on my due date. Adam had arrived two weeks early, and I expected to go early this time around, too, but no such luck. I was only ten percent effaced, and one centimeter dilated. I headed home to wait.

As days turned into weeks, I became more uncomfortable, and Rod and I were worried about the baby. At the nine-and-a-half month appointment, as soon as the doctor opened the exam room door, I announced that no matter what happened that night I'd be coming to the hospital the next morning to be induced.

"Yes, we'll plan for an induction tomorrow morning. Get there by seven, and we'll begin the Pitocin drip." Pitocin is synthetic oxytocin, the hormone that induces labor.

That's all I needed to hear. I was ready for this baby to be born!

On the way back to the car, Rod said, laughing, "I feared for that doctor's life if he told you to come back in a few more days."

"That was not an option!"

I woke up extra early, got a quick shower, and headed downstairs to give Adam his breakfast. "You'll be a big brother, soon," I told him. Once Rod loaded the car, we headed to my parents' house, where we gave Adam a big brother gift—Mr. and Mrs. Potato Head—to play with while we were gone.

"Good luck!" Mom said. "Pretty soon we'll be holding our little granddaughter."

"I think we're right. Sarah Morgan will be here soon!"

Once we checked in, I was taken upstairs in a wheelchair. The nurses were friendly, and the check-in process was uneventful. Within no time, the doctor began induction, and the nurse kept an eye on me. Just around noon, the pain intensified, and I reminded them about the epidural. When the anesthesiologist came an hour later, he moved me into position and took out his syringe. Rod, who was trying to comfort me, took one look at the syringe, and fainted, all six foot six of him falling to the floor. The nurse must have seen this before. She knelt at his side, thrust smelling salts up to his nose, then helped him to the chair.

"Sorry honey, I just got a little dizzy," Rod said, still dazed.

I remained upright as the anesthesiologist finished and the medicine took effect. Then I announced, "I'm going to throw up, and I have to push."

The nurse at my side passed me an emesis basin and said, "Do not push till you're in the delivery room."

The delivery room was very cold. I trembled from head to toe and my teeth chattered due to the rush of hormones and adrenaline. I was near exhaustion. A very enthusiastic nurse coached me through the pushing, but after an hour, I was exhausted and my pushes were ineffective. I heard the doctor mumble something about a c-section. Rod leaned into my right ear and said, "Honey you have to push really hard.

You're almost there. Just a little longer, but if you don't get the baby out soon, they're going to do a c-section. So, push!"

On the very next attempt, I gave it my all and out came our seven-pound, eight-ounce little girl.

When Adam visited late that afternoon, he was sweet with his little sister. He kept saying, "She is so adorable," every time his gaze met hers.

We went home two days later. I was glad that Adam was already potty trained. It would have been difficult, as well as expensive, to have both children in diapers at the same time. Adam helped out by getting diapers or onesies for baby Sarah. He became very protective of his little sister. Whenever relatives or friends stopped by, Adam watched them like a hawk when they were holding Sarah. Sometimes he'd sit very close to her in case she needed him. I'd often see him standing by the bassinette, talking to her or watching her sleep. It was adorable to watch.

There was a new commercial about Estee Lauder and the jingle was so catchy it kept playing in my head. At one point, I added Sarah's name to the jungle.

I'd sing loudly, "Sarah Morgan Estee Lauder." Then Rod and I would giggle. It was a catchy tune we'd both sing from time to time.

One day, we were in the car driving when Adam heard the commercial on the radio. He said, puzzled, "That's my Estee Lauder. Why are they talking about my sister on the radio?"

"Estee Lauder is the name of a company," I explained. "I added baby Sarah's name to the song because it sounded so cute."

"Don't worry baby Sarah," he said, patting her arm. "You belong to me, not the people on the radio."

CHAPTER 18

LIFE IS GOOD

I loved being a mom to my two little ones. I always had a lot to juggle, but I was fortunate to have a mom and dad who loved my children as much as we did and were ready to jump in when we needed them.

I typically worked the evening or night shift. I also signed up with a nursing agency, through which I was assigned to many different facilities, usually in the ICU or CCU, and could potentially make more money. For a time I was the assigned nursing supervisor for a nursing home. I never minded change. I grew up in a military family, where we moved at the drop of a hat. I always found learning new procedures and routines to be challenging and exciting, never intimidating or overwhelming.

I enrolled Adam in preschool at the Wyomissing Institute of Fine Arts. He thrived at the institute. After one look at the ballet studio, with the mirrors and barre, he was in! He took ballet for one semester, and he did really well at the year-end performance, surrounded by all his girlfriends, as he called them. He stayed at the institute through kindergarten before moving to public school at Breaknock Elementary for first grade, where he was placed in their gifted program.

When Sarah was old enough, she also attended the institute. She was always the social butterfly in her class, and thrived there as well. She went to kindergarten at Breaknock, though, because her big brother was already there.

Then one day Rod came home from Cartech with exciting news. He had been contacted by a headhunter, who wanted him to interview for Vice President at a copper stamping company, Ansonia Copper and Brass in Ansonia, Connecticut. He was flattered and excited.

I said, "What the heck, it couldn't hurt to interview."

He drove four hours to Ansonia for an interview with George Wilson, the president of the company. The two hit it off immediately and within a short time, he received an offer. He would start in the role of VP and a year later, when the president retired, Rod would take over as president. His salary would be more than twice what he was making, plus a yearly bonus.

I told Rod we had to make the move, but he got cold feet. He liked the job, but he wasn't sure about moving away from his aging family. I had moved so many times in my life, it wasn't a big deal to me. I finally said, "Rod we have to do this for our children. This is closer to New York City. Think of the culture! Think of the opportunities. Let's pray about it, but I believe the Lord is opening another door, so don't be afraid to walk through it."

"How am I going to tell my family?"

"With honesty. I have to do the same thing. The kids will love it."

We arranged an exploratory trip to check out Southbury, the town George Wilson recommended we live in. I told my parents why we were going to Connecticut, but Rod wanted to wait until we knew for sure.

Our realtor, Gordon, gave us a tour of the town first. I found Southbury to be an absolutely lovely part of the country, inviting and charming, a great place to raise a family. The school system was exceptional.

Gordon took us to look at houses on Saturday afternoon. As the afternoon progressed, he showed us nicer but also more expensive houses. It was late afternoon when we found "the One," at least for me. The outside of the house was gray cedar clapboard, with black shutters and a black front door. It had a cute covered front porch, and tall trees shading the house in the front yard. Around the side was a garage with three bays, which Rod loved. The yard had plenty of room for flower-beds I could get my hands dirty in. Inside, the first story floors were a burnished hardwood. A wooden stairway of white trim and decorative crown molding curved upstairs from the foyer. In the dining room, the China cabinets were set off by classic columns, also white, and the kitchen cabinets, white again, were tall and spacious, with the teal countertops providing a pop of color. Another stairway ascended from the den to the four bedrooms upstairs.

Rod took Gordon aside and said, "Kim has fallen in love with this house. Is there any way we can afford it?"

"Let's go to my office and run some numbers."

In the end, Rod took the job, we bought the house, and we moved. Rod's family was disappointed, but they understood. Rod's salary was well more than our combined salary had been in Pennsylvania, and that was hard to turn down. That Rod was going to take over as president was a big draw as well. This is why we decided I would stay at home at least for a while, even though the cost of living was higher in Southbury—to get us settled and take care of the children, who were six and eight by then.

I was in a constant state of awe and gratitude knowing this was all ours.

Culturally, we now lived in the hub, and we wanted to take full advantage. We took the train from the Southeast Station in Brewster, New York, into the city. We went to plays and musicals and dined at the 21 Club as often as possible. We ventured into Chinatown, where we found the best knock-offs and great food. In Little Italy, the rich smell of espresso drew us into the bakeries where we bought tiramisu, cannoli, and coffee. Christmas was our favorite time to go into the city, when it was transformed into a spectacular winter wonderland.

We waited in line to see the department store windows with their animated themes—Santa's Workshop, Toyland, the Nutcracker—and we went to the Rockettes' holiday performance every year.

The kids loved their new school, the neighborhood, and the new friends they made. They joined soccer and basketball, where Rod and I coached some of their teams. Before we moved, we had sold Rod's car to purchase a shiny ebony baby grand so the kids could take piano lessons. For exercise, we ran on the bridle paths with our Weimaraner, Madison. We were moving on up.

I became room mom for both kids' classrooms and served on the PTO at Pomperaug Elementary School with my new friend Judy. Then one day a brief discussion with the school nurse led me to a part-time position there as school nurse. This was 1996. It was exciting to work at the kids' school. I got to know many more children and families from the area.

Life was good.

But I always had this underlying shame, this feeling that I didn't deserve to be happy because of what had happened when I was thirteen. The PTSD never quite went away and manifested itself at the strangest times and places. If you had asked me if I ever would have harmed myself, I would have answered an emphatic, "Not a chance." As a Christian, I don't believe anyone should commit suicide. It has always been a strong conviction of mine, instilled since childhood. It's giving up on God.

Yet one morning I considered doing just that—taking my own life.

It was one of those perfectly normal mornings. Breakfast as usual then off to our daughter's first grade classroom. Ever since Sarah graduated from Arizona State University, and as soon as my fingerprint background check returned from our state, I started volunteering in her classroom as needed. I always had fun volunteering, and that day the children were as cute as ever. I oversaw arts and crafts, helped with cutting and gluing, then clean-up. I hugged Sarah good-bye and headed home as her classroom walked to lunch.

I pulled up to a traffic light that had just turned red. With my left turn signal on, I idled and waited for the light to change. I wasn't thinking about anything important, when suddenly my mind was seized by a powerful voice: *Pull out in front of the fastest cars and end your pain now! You don't have to put up with it anymore. Everyone will think it was an accident. Wait. Those cars are too slow. Hers are two good ones, much faster. Get ready to step on the gas.* But the light changed, and the oncoming car slowed to a stop.

I snapped back to reality, trembling and upset. *Where did* that *come from? It's a good morning! I've never felt like that before! I came this close* .... The desire to end my life had been very intense for those few seconds. I had had these kinds of intrusive thoughts before, but never to kill myself. I called my counselor as soon as I got home and saw her the next day. We had much more work to do.

A poem, Confidences,[4] by my friend Shelley Kitchura Nelson captures that day for me.

Confidences
Shelley J. Kitchura Nelson

Between the two of us the road is dark; still,
It shines like a night lake in the moon's light.
Gray surrounds it.
Sitting in the driver's seat we feel what comes up
from the black in what we imagine is our fate.
Two separate instances, both out of control.
You think of how easy it would be to step on the gas—
remove the pain instantly.
I push the gas pedal and think of the lake—
Either way it's a long thought.
By then the road has brought us home and
the seconds are gone and our families don't know.
You trust that God has made this plan.

I'm not sure what to believe,
except that the plan isn't working.
The dogs and our houses are happy to see
you there, me here.

✦ ✦ ✦

There was another hiccup in our otherwise perfect life, this one Rod's. At Rod's year mark on the job, George, the president of the company, told Rod he wasn't retiring after all, that he had a few more good years left in him. This was in violation of Rod's contract.

Rod came home from work that day defeated and disappointed. You could argue that it wasn't that big a deal, that the president would retire eventually, that Rod should just ride it out. He liked the job as vice president, didn't he?

He did until he didn't. The problem was, the union employees hated George as president and couldn't wait until Rod took over. When they made their views known to the board, George grew angry and took it out on Rod, making his life miserable with corporate politics—all of a sudden, everything that went well was George's doing, and everything that went badly was Rod's. Rod now hated every minute of his job and became so stressed at night he'd wake from a nightmare into a full-blown panic attack.

Although he was under stress, he did a good job of not taking it out on me and the kids. He continued being a loving Dad and supportive coach, and he still rubbed my back at night until I fell asleep. He was always such a tender and romantic man.

Rod got in touch with the headhunter, who sent him on interviews throughout Pennsylvania and Connecticut. He almost took a position as president of a steel mill in western Pennsylvania, until we actually visited the town and saw that it was stuck in the fifties. Culturally, we had gotten used to being near the City. We weren't ready to change that.

Rod ended up taking a vice-president job at a German-owned metal fabrication company in Waterbury, Connecticut. It was a lateral move, but the commute was actually shorter than the one to Ansonia and we wouldn't have to move!

After three years of working as a nurse for the Region 15 School District, in 1999, a full-time job opened across Main Street at Gainfield Elementary School. I had worked there many times, and the fulltime nurse, Elaine Kahn, had asked me to apply.

I spoke with Rod, and the kids before putting my name in for the job. Once I did, I received the offer. Before accepting, though, I wanted to talk to the principal, John Mudry, about an emergency plan.

"Why do we need an emergency plan?" he asked when we sat down in his office.

"It's common sense. We need to know we can get all the children to safety in an emergency. I'm a critical care nurse and used to dealing with emergencies, but no one else here has that training."

"We've never had an emergency we couldn't handle."

"John, I'm a critical care nurse. I know what can happen. I won't work here unless you let me develop an emergency plan—which we will practice monthly, by the way."

He rubbed his face while he was thinking. "Okay," he said.

"Thank you. I'll work on it on the beach over the summer."

I drew a sigh of relief. *Thank God John believes in me.*

I wasn't kidding about writing the plan on the beach. Even before I met Rod, I had always loved the Jersey Shore, particularly Cape May and the barrier islands, and of course the shore played a role in getting Rod and me together. We tried to go there every summer, no matter where we were living. That summer was going to be special, however. It was the first summer we'd stay in our own place, a twin house on a barrier island off of the coast of New Jersey that we got each other as a 20th anniversary present in 1999.

A twin house meant that we shared a wall with our neighbors, though we each owned the land our units were built on. Our neighbors were great, though, so that was never a problem.

This house was our retreat, one we could use no matter the season. It was just a short walk to the private beach, where we hung out with our beach friends, as we called them, who liked to sit next to us for our music and general friendliness. We had a huge beach cart to haul our boom box and CDs as well our cooler, chairs, towels, blankets, sports equipment, and boogie boards. The kids had to carry their own surf boards, though. The cart wasn't *that* big.

Rod didn't have the luxury of summers off, so he came down from Connecticut on the weekends, then got on the road Monday morning at three-fifteen and conducted business with the Germans for most of his four-hour commute. They were impressed with his dedication and the fact that he was awake so early.

When you have a beach house, you always get plenty of summer guests. Like my mom, though, I loved to entertain, and guests were never a problem for me. My parents, Rod's mom and grandparents, his dad and stepmother, Cee, other family members, and many friends came to visit that summer and many after. The kids especially enjoyed having their friends from Connecticut come down. We loved showing everyone around the town and boardwalk, a timeless slice of American life we felt privileged to be part of.

We had a four-passenger jet ski that we took on many adventures. Just about everyone enjoyed taking a ride out into the bay, which was generally calm. Those who were a bit more fearless, however, I'd take out into the open ocean where we rode the untamed waves like bronco busters, then I'd turn off the engine and float to see what we could see. Once my friend Heather and I found ourselves sitting in the middle of a massive school of pink rays, I had swum with and even kissed a gray ray while in Bora Bora with Sarah, but we had never seen pink ones!

We held our breath and watched them silently as they frolicked in the water around us. Talk about witnessing God's grandeur! Another time my passenger and I ended up in a pod of curious dolphins. I was going to dive in and swim with the dolphins until we noticed that there were females with their calves. You don't mess with a female and her calves, whatever the species! I left it for another time.

In addition to all the beach fun, I worked every day on Gainfield's evacuation plan. I didn't want to forget anything. If the emergency hit during recess, many children could be in far off fields. I'd need a bag full of emergency supplies so I could run to any location quickly. We'd also need to be able to clear the school's entire premises in the case of a bomb threat. I talked with John by phone, and he told me we could take the children to the back of the school and across the street, where there was a large area for everyone to stand that was far enough from the school. We'd also need an emergency team to help me carry my equipment and get people safely to the local hospitals. John agreed that we should practice monthly, just as we did fire drills. I thought I had it down.

At the end of our fun-filled summer, we returned to Connecticut for the new school year. Rod was happy to have us home. I started school ahead of the children for orientation as a new hire. When I finally got the keys to my office, I reorganized the office and infirmary, cleaned out the cabinets, tossed some things, hung new pictures, and propped open the door, ready for business.

CHAPTER 19

AN UNSETTLING TIME

The fall in New England was always spectacular with the leaves in full brilliance in the brightest of golds, burgundy, and orange. In the mornings a dense fog covered the ground. The air outside was crisp, although the earth was still warm. Pine trees dotted the hills and valleys, while the massive maples were rigged with spouts to drain the thick, sweet sap into waiting buckets for cooking into the amber maple syrup sold in every gift shop in the northeast.

The snow started early that year and the kids always prayed for snow days off from school. Some days their prayers were answered, but on others they were grumpy with disappointment when I woke them and they had to go to school. Sarah and I both got cross-country skis for Christmas that year and Adam got a snowboard. The kids loved to go to the small ski slope in Woodbury, one town north of us. When they weren't playing outside, they huddled by our fireplace, drinking hot cocoa and miniature marshmallows.

Rod was very busy at work, flying over 100,000 miles each year to set up plants in China and Europe. It was taking its toll. All that travel was physically exhausting, but he also didn't care for the extended periods away from us. Our kids were growing up quickly, and he hated missing the milestones. He didn't particularly care for life in New England, either. Even after several years, he found it too upscale, and he missed his family back home.

When he wasn't traveling, Rod coached both kids in basketball, while I kept score at their games. Sarah was on an AAU team, and Adam was on the school team—until he fractured his forearm during a game. By the sound of his primal groan and a mother's intuition, I immediately knew something was wrong. I ran out on the court joined by a doctor from the stands. The doctor—a gynecologist, mind you—said Adam was fine, probably just a bruise. But he was pale and sweating heavily and guarding his arm gingerly. I knew in a second it was fractured, no matter what the gynecologist said. Within a few hours, Adam was in a cast in the ER at the Waterbury Hospital.

We had put the children in a private school, St. Margaret McTernan in Waterbury, which was highly regarded for the quality of its academics and the beauty of its campus, with its acres of rolling hills. Rod could take the kids to school in the morning, and when he was traveling, they could get the bus at the commuter lot. Adam thrived in his classes, but sociable Sarah disliked the small classes and restrictive uniforms.

"Please let me go back to Rochambeau," she begged one night at dinner. Rochambeau was the public middle school. "I hate St. Margaret's."

"St. Margaret's is a great school, Sarah. And we've already paid your tuition for the year," I said.

"It's not a great school for *me*," she said. "My class has ten kids in it, and they're all nerds!"

"Stop talking like that," I corrected her sternly.

"Dad," she said, trying a different tack. "Come to school. You'll see."

"Okay," he said. "That's fair. But Mom's right. You'll probably have to stay for the year."

Later that week, Rod visited the school and attended lunch with the kids in their formal dining room, where tables were set with white tablecloths, cloth napkins, and all the correct silverware, properly placed.

I couldn't wait to hear what Rod had to say that night. I grabbed him before dinner, without the kids around. "Well?"

"She's right!"

"What?"

"Her class is tiny, and they spew privilege. Sarah must feel like a caged animal. I think she'll be happier at Rochambeau, I really do."

She was ecstatic when Rod told her.

"YES! Thank you. Thank you. Thank you, Dad. I can't wait to tell my friends."

Time moved along, as it does.

Since taking the full-time nurse role, I wasn't able to attend the Southbury Garden Club meetings. I missed my friends and our projects. The herb garden I spearheaded at The Bend of River Audubon had been well received, and I missed getting my bare hands into soil and then sitting back to watch the flowers poke their little heads above ground.

Rod had begun running. We ran together with Madison on the weekends on the scenic bridle paths. We had to keep an eye on Madison because she liked to eat the horse droppings, but we were usually too late to stop her. Sometimes, despite their groans of protest, we made the kids ride their bikes with us while we ran. I'd like to think they remember those times fondly. I know I do. It was a more innocent time.

Each summer, the kids and I returned to our barrier island home in Wildwood, where they got better and better at longboard surfing. I stuck to the boogie board, which I used whenever I ventured into the deeper, murky water. Rod continued to work during the week and drive down on weekends, though year after year he grew increasingly dissatisfied with living and working in Connecticut. It got to the point where he talked about purchasing a business in the Reading area and moving back to simplify things. He already had a business in mind.

This was an unsettling time for me. I wanted Rod to be happy, but I also wanted the kids to be happy. I knew the kids loved Connecticut and wouldn't want to move. I'm a people pleaser. This is the kind of situation that makes a people pleaser's head explode—the risk of disappointing one or the other of someone she loves. At the same time, we were still the parents, and we would make the decision for all of us.

While all this was weighing on my mind, I still had a job to do. I arrived for work and opened my office door as usual. Because it was the only bathroom on this side of the building, my co-workers often used the bathroom in my back office.

Cyndie, one of the paraprofessionals, walked in my office to use the bathroom, I assumed, but stopped at my desk. "You look drained! Are you okay?"

"Yeah," I said. "Just a lot going on at home."

"Why don't you come in early tomorrow? I'll do some energy work on you. You might feel better."

I didn't really know what energy work was. Cyndie was a little intuitive, but I was willing to go along. "Okay, what do I have to do?" I asked.

"Nothing. Just show up early. I'll do the rest."

The next morning, Cyndie had me lie down on one of the infirmary beds. "Close your eyes and relax, I won't even touch you," she instructed. "You might feel a bit different afterwards, a little sad or silly, but it passes quickly."

I closed my eyes and drifted a bit. Several minutes passed. I saw vivid colors against my eyelids. Lime green, hot pink, bright teal, a burst of orange and bright yellow. "Why am I seeing so many bright colors?"

"We'll talk about that."

She continued. I giggled.

"What?" Cyndie asked.

"I feel like I have the biggest horse teeth in my mouth. They're so big I can't close my lips."

"That's the silliness I was talking about."

I giggled a little more, then calmed down.

She worked in silence for a while, then said, "I have a message for you from someone that passed. Is that okay?"

"I guess," I said.

"I'm not understanding her name. Something like, Emmie. No, that's not quite it. Ellie, no I'm not saying it correctly."

"Is it Evey?" I suggested.

"Evey, yes, it's Evey! She wants me to tell you she will be with you."

I opened my eyes and sat up. "My Aunt Evey was killed in a car accident several years ago. My dad's sister. That's a strange message. Is that all she said?"

"Yes."

Then I laid down again and Cyndie continued. Within a short time, I started laughing hysterically.

"What's so funny?"

"As best as I could between laughter, I explained that I felt like I had a set of horse teeth in my mouth. The teeth seemed so large that I felt like I could no longer close my mouth over them." And the laughter continued.

"I can do another session anytime. I hope that helped."

"Thanks, Cyndie. I'm going to laugh every time I think about those horse teeth."

This took place several days before the accident. When I thought about it afterwards, I was sure Aunt Evey knew what was about to happen. Some things are without explanation, and this was one of them.

Rod had made one trip to Pennsylvania to scout out the business he wanted to buy and took a second after my session with Cyndie to look more deeply into the business's finances. This was on May 1, 2002. He was returning from that trip the day of my accident. The day life changed for us all.

PART IV

································

FALLOUT FROM THE ACCIDENT

"All I knew for sure was that I was tired and empty."

—*Joan Anderson,*
A Year by the Sea:
Thoughts of an Unfinished Woman[5]

CHAPTER 20

A NIGHT OF TRAUMA SURGERY

While my life hung in the balance in the OR, Rod found his way to the waiting room and prepared himself for a long night of waiting, wondering, and worrying. He was joined in his vigil by my principal, John Mudry; by one of the nurses I worked with, Maureen Feeney; and the Director of Special Education Services, Donna Popowski. They offered prayers and kind words, but nothing took away Rod's fear of losing me. He spoke with both children and assured them I was at the best hospital in Connecticut. He told Carole he thought Sarah should go on the class trip the next day, that it would be a good diversion.

Once scrubbed and gowned, Dr. Yue entered the operating room where several of his residents were waiting to give him a quick update. All the x-rays as well as the CT scans were within view. The right leg had sustained the most fractures while the left leg had lost the most muscle. In my lower right leg and foot, I had fourteen compound fractures—fractures so severe the bone protruded from the skin. In addition, seven centimeters of bone near the ankle had been pulverized and was missing and the Achilles tendon had ruptured. An area near the inner right ankle would require cadaver skin grafting.

The lower left leg sustained two compound fractures, and that Achilles tendon had torn as well. The biggest challenge on the left leg was that ninety percent of the calf muscle had been torn off and there was a large gaping wound on the back of my lower leg. The doctors surmised that over the previous six hours, without tourniquets around my legs, I had lost half of my blood supply. That was why I had lost consciousness and why my blood pressure was critically low.

Dr. Yue knew time was critical. He decided to begin surgery on the right leg after placing a tourniquet around the left. He asked the anesthesiologist to give me as much blood, blood products, and intravenous fluids as possible as quickly as possible. If they had followed my request for no blood products, I wouldn't have made it through surgery.

When the surgery on the right leg was completed, if my blood pressure was stable enough to remove the tourniquet from the left leg, Dr. Yue would start surgery on that leg. To stabilize the fractures while they healed, I required a specialized external fixator on both my legs. These devices were to be bolted to my bones from the outside of the skin. After the fractures had healed, I would need to regrow the seven centimeters of bone I had lost.

The first surgery took many hours. The anesthesiologist was able to give me twelve units of blood, multiple units of blood products, and many liters of IV fluid.

When Dr. Yue had finished, he asked if my blood pressure was stable, and he was given the okay to remove the left leg tourniquet and operate. With only ten percent of the calf muscle intact and viable, Dr. Yue fileted the muscle in half to cover as much of the posterior calf as possible, since the opening encompassed an area from the mid-calf to the ankle. He knew he would have to talk with a plastic surgeon in the morning to manage the left leg after he finished.

The sun was just beginning to rise in the eastern sky when I was wheeled out of the operating room and taken to the Intensive Care Unit. That's where I was when I first opened my eyes. I became immediately aware of extraordinary pain and extreme nausea from the anesthesia and the narcotics. I was very happy to see Rod, but I dozed on and off throughout the day between intense periods of pain, vomiting, and dry heaving. At times I was delirious from the mix of intense pain and narcotics. When the nurse brought food into my room, the mere smell brought on more vomiting.

Several parents from the elementary school visited briefly, but I was too sick to talk to them. No one told me at that time, but I had third-spaced the fluid they had given me in the operating room because of how much and how quickly it had been administered. When you third-space fluid, the fluid seeps out of your blood vessels and into the surrounding tissue, so a person appears to be very swollen everywhere. My face was puffy, my eyes were swollen, and my fingers were so swollen it hurt to bend them. Even my arms and legs were twice their normal size. I was almost unrecognizable. It didn't really matter, though, because I knew that in a few days the extra fluid would be reabsorbed, and my body would return to normal. In fact, I should have been grateful. That huge volume of fluid and blood had likely saved my life.

My feet were elevated with many pillows, and I could see cobalt blue metal fixators attached to my lower legs. The vigil at my bedside was the same whenever I opened my eyes. Rod held my hand and offered encouragement. He stayed at my bedside around the clock. It was especially comforting to know that if I was too sick to advocate for myself, he'd step in for me. I tried not to think about the road ahead, but when I thought about it, I realized the Angel had taken all my fear away. I no longer feared anything, really. Eleanor Roosevelt once said, "The purpose of life is to live it, to taste experience to the utmost, to reach out eagerly and without fear, for newer and richer experiences."[6] I wonder if Angels visited her as well.

Over the next few days, when I wasn't in surgery or pain, vomiting, or sleeping (more like passed out), I thought about the beautiful, prayerful visitor in the ambulance the Lord had sent to ease my fear and pain. I was humbled that He thought enough of me to give me such peace, the kind I had never experienced before. I had a tough time wrapping my head around that peace, what it meant. After I prayed about it for several days, the Lord helped me out. He told me to think of it as The Peace That Passes All Understanding. *The peace that passes all understanding*, I pondered. *Am I really that special to Him?* It felt amazingly, well, peaceful to linger in those thoughts. *I certainly will never be afraid of dying again.*

Fear is not of God. Fear is a device of the enemy designed to side-track us from focusing on God. God fills our hearts with peace and love, which cancels fear. This is why we are to put our trust in God; because His guidance will never give us reason to fear. I thanked Him, because I no longer had reason to doubt, fear, or fret, because His peace would always be with me. I could strike fear and worry from my vocabulary.

But the Lord sends us trials as well. These beautiful thoughts abruptly ended when excruciating pain jolted through me, intensifying by the second. Several weeks passed before I was able to think again about that peace that passes all understanding. That kind of peace would be hard to come by for a long, long time.

CHAPTER 21

SURGERY, PAIN, PUKE, REPEAT

D r. Joseph Shin, Head of Plastic and Reconstructive Surgery, and several of his residents visited me to evaluate and treat the wound on my left leg. He determined that I required debridement surgery the following day to remove unviable tissue to prevent complications. Shortly after, an anesthesiologist visited to interview me in preparation for the next surgery. Early the next morning, I was taken to the OR for the debridement. When I woke up from the anesthesia, once again, the combination of anesthesia and narcotics made for an awful day of nausea and dizziness.

In the middle of the second night, a nurse woke me to let me know I was being transferred to another nursing unit. She told me that a massive remodel of the ICU was beginning in several hours, and the unit would be closed until completion. She assured me that I would still be monitored closely since they were sending me to a telemetry unit, staffed by critical care nurses. Within minutes all my wound supplies and belongings were packed, and I was en route to another floor. I was placed in another large private room. A cot as well as linens was brought to the room for Rod to sleep on. I'm sure that was better than the chair he had slept on in the ICU, although I was certain that most cots were not made for men as tall as he is.

Surgery continued every day as the gaping wound on the back of my left calf required daily debridement to keep infection at bay. I was told that I'd eventually require a skin graft. More surgeries meant more anesthesia and more narcotics, which meant more pain, nausea, and vomiting. Food gagged me, and I didn't even want to see it, smell it, or hear about it. I was losing a great deal of weight, but no one really noticed since there was so much else going on. Most days the pain was so intense, despite all the pain medication, that I seldom spoke. It was easier to stay quiet as I suffered. Rod didn't need to know how bad it was. I've heard it said that bone pain is the most intense kind of pain, and I can verify that. When I did get a brief respite from the pain and fell asleep from sheer exhaustion, I knew that I would wake up when the pain came back. I didn't get much sleep. I woke up on my back with my legs hanging painfully in their barbaric cages. I moved to the right, *No try the left*, I'd tell myself, but repositioning my legs gave me no relief. I gently rubbed my thighs, hoping that a distraction above the site of the pain would make a difference, but nothing changed.

There was another problem with the narcotics I had to take to get through every day. I was in recovery from alcohol addiction, and I was afraid I would replace one addiction with another. I had worked too hard to let it all go! But then my pain would set in, and all bets were off! There was a always a battle raging inside me. Many times it was so intense I prayed silently for the Lord to take me home, but then I'd look into the eyes of my husband and small children, and I knew I had to keep fighting.

Sarah enjoyed her three-day class trip to Boston, the perfect diversion for our social butterfly. She returned on Friday evening. Adam continued to stay with Ryan's family, attending school daily. On Friday, Heather, my teacher friend and running partner, picked him up at the bus stop after school and brought him to the hospital for his first visit. It was good to finally see him. I sensed that he needed to see me in one piece again.

By the third day my wider family suddenly started showing up at the hospital, much to my surprise. First my parents, then my brothers and their wives, then my nieces and nephews, and last my stepson, all traveling from other states. I was so happy to see them, and it gave me a great deal of comfort to know they were all here and could help out Rod and the kids. Because of the severe pain, though, I wasn't great company and couldn't really hold a conversation. They all seemed to understand.

What no one told me was that the doctors had told Rod there was still a good chance I wouldn't survive, that at some point I likely would develop an infection that would travel through my bones and kill me. This could happen any time in the first three months. No wonder everyone rushed to Connecticut to get one last opportunity to spend time with me.

After the fourth surgery, I was transferred to the orthopedic unit, which was on the seventh floor. I remained there for the next three-and-a-half months, but I'm glad I didn't know that at the time. Sometimes ignorance is, if not bliss, then at least a small mercy.

Sometime after I was transferred to the orthopedic unit at Yale Hospital, Officer Don came by to take a sworn statement. I was surprised to see him so soon—I thought they'd give me a little more time to recover, but they have their jobs to do as well. I introduced him to Rod, whom I asked to stay. It would be the first time I discussed the accident.

I started from the moment I pulled into the parking lot at Denmo's. As I spoke, I began to tremble. At first, it was just a mild shaking, but before I got to the point of impact, my teeth were chattering. Rod asked me if I was cold. I told him I wasn't, but by the end of the interview, my entire body was violently quaking from head to toe. Rod went to get the nurse, and when they returned, the nurse put her hand on my arm and looked at Officer Don, who wrapped it up quickly after that. I felt sheepish. I was a critical care nurse! I should have been able to give a statement without falling apart. This was just one of many indications that things were going to get harder before they got easier.

The staff members were all wonderful, caring people, who went above and beyond duty to make my experience as seamless as possible. I will forever hold a special place in my heart for them. They were competent and professional, yet they also listened to me when I cried out in pain and frustration. They encouraged me when I felt like giving up and gave me hope amid pain and confusion.

For continuity of care, I typically had the same nurse and aides assigned to me. The RNs included Brooke and Christina. Joe was my orderly, Megan was my physical therapist, and Debbie was an LPN or nurse's aide.

I will never forget how Debbie prayed. She came up with beautiful, spontaneous, and personal prayers that gave me a profound sense of peace. About halfway through each one, she would break into language I had never heard before. I think she was speaking in tongues! I always wondered what she was saying. All I know is that she uplifted me time and time again. She was such a sweet and beautiful Christian woman. I felt so blessed to know her during those horrific days and nights.

Because of how long I was hospitalized, my family also developed a good rapport with the staff members. They, too, would confide in them when times got difficult, and the staff was wonderful about listening and offering solutions when they could.

As you can imagine after such a tragic accident the news spread quickly throughout our small New England towns. Within days of the accident, people from Southbury, Woodbury, Waterbury, and other nearby towns did incredible acts of kindness for our family. They dropped off prepared meals, sometimes three to four per day. Others bought gift certificates to local restaurants near our home as well as restaurants in the New Haven area near the hospital. They helped us tremendously, and we were very grateful. Words could never fully express our gratitude.

My extended family did make one big mistake, though. Since so many family members visited the hospital each day and stayed for long periods of time, they decided to bring crockpots to the hospital so they could have hot food when they were hungry. Electrical items from home are a no-no at a hospital. The risk of fire is too great. Well, my family didn't realize this, and I was out of it, so I had no clue that they were setting up a daily buffet of heated foods in the waiting room—until the staff found out and sent the crockpots home.

By Sunday, my parents, brothers, sisters in law, nieces, and nephews said goodbye and returned to their homes. My stepson Jason stayed longer than the others and was very supportive while he was there. He helped out so his dad could get a shower and shave every once in a while. I was truly blessed to have such an amazing family and friends.

CHAPTER 22

MORE MESSENGERS

Yet another surgery was scheduled for late morning. It was always nice when the kids could see me off. The nurse checked my bracelet, my chart was in order, and transport had just arrived. I kissed Rod, Sarah, and Adam, then we each did the "I love you" sign. All available staff came in, helped lift me onto the litter, and then covered me with blankets. I was whisked without delay down the long corridors towards the operating room.

My heart pounded with anxiety. I felt safe in the confines of the hospital room with its trained staff who knew how to take care of the fixators holding my legs in place. Once I left the room, I grew agitated and paranoid, fearful of reinjuring my legs. I went into hypervigilant mode, nervously looking from side to side in anticipation of danger. My heart pounded. I perspired profusely. I watched the litter as it was maneuvered around wheelchairs and other obstacles. I caught sight of my legs, and slipped into a kind of hallucinatory flashback to the time just after the accident. *Oh my God, help me. They're going to fall off! My legs are severed and going to fall off. They are swinging like a pendulum, then twisting and turning out of control. Please help me*

Lord, my legs are going to fall off. God Help Me! Why do I keep seeing my severed legs?

When I finally was pushed into the operating room, the familiar sound of Shep's voice snapped me back to reality. I felt as if I had reached another safe zone. Shep was the anesthetist I had gotten to know. He had been a medic in Vietnam, and I was certain he had seen injuries like mine all the time. Maybe that's why he had taken an interest in me. He also knew that I had spent fifteen years as a critical care nurse so we could discuss the medical aspects of my case. On days I didn't have surgery, he visited me to see how I was doing.

"Hi Shep. Always good to see you."

"When you're on the schedule, I'll always take care of you."

"That's comforting to know!" I looked around the sterile, bright, cool room where all familiar faces smiled at me. It felt like home. Even the clanging of instruments comforted me as my racing heart finally slowed down. I took a deep, cleansing breath of operating room air and slowly released it as my litter came to rest next to the OR table. I crossed my arms over my chest as they lifted me onto the operating table.

I always helped Shep at this point, so I unsnapped my gown as he reached in and applied the heart monitor leads. Next, I extended my index finger for the pulse oximeter. The nurses had already placed the boards on either side of my arms, so I extended my left arm for the Velcro straps that held my arm in place. Shep let me to hold the mask with my other hand while he administered the anesthesia. Once I was asleep, my right arm would be strapped on the arm board as well.

Dr. Shin entered the OR and approached the table to make sure everything was prepped for him.

Shep handed me the oxygen mask. "Ready?"

"Yep." I breathed through the mask. The voices faded and the room closed in as I gently closed my eyes for another surgery.

+ + +

During one such operation early in the process, Rod and the boys—Adam and Jason, who was still in town—were famished, so they decided to eat lunch in the cafeteria. Since there were many different stations, Rod gave each boy some cash and told them to meet up at a table once they all had their food. Adam and Jason quickly found prepared foods and met at the register. After they paid, they found an empty table and sat down. Rod had decided on something that needed to be cooked so his meal took a bit longer. The boys had only been sitting for a few minutes. They were already eating and talking when an elderly, disheveled, poorly dressed Black man who appeared homeless sat down at their table with some food. He did not make eye contact, nor did he speak. He just quietly ate.

After Rod paid for his food, he spotted the boys and joined them at the table. "Why are we sitting here? We can't talk privately." Before they could answer, the stranger raised his head and spoke directly to them. "I know that you are all very upset, but I've come to tell you that she's going to be okay. There is one member of your family who isn't here today. She is a good basketball player." He made eye contact with Adam and said, "Because of this, you are going to do amazing things with your life. You are also having some issues with a girl but don't worry about that any longer."

No one moved or made a sound. Then he spoke to Jason. "You have no idea how important you are to your family, and it is good that you are here to support everyone during this difficult time. Most important though is that you all realize that she is going to be okay." After he said his piece, he got out of his seat, pushed his chair in, bussed his tray, and walked out the door.

Rod told me later that he and the two boys sat in silence for several minutes, and that every time he went to the cafeteria in the next three and a half months, he tried to find this man again, but he never did. This was their Angel moment. The man was sent to deliver this message of hope when they needed it most.

During another surgery on a gorgeous late spring day, sunny but not too hot, Rod and the kids—this time Adam and Sarah—decided to go outside and get lunch. Every day numerous food vendors set up on the green across the street.

They headed to the elevator and once inside, Sarah pressed 1. The elevator came to a stop on the fourth floor and a middle-aged man entered and pressed 2. As soon as the doors closed, the man turned to face the three of them. "I just want to assure you that she is going to be okay." By the time he had finished, the doors had opened and he turned around and left. The doors closed. The three stood there speechless, and when the doors opened again, they walked out of the elevator and remained silent until they were outside. The same thing had happened before. Another time Rod and the kids were in the elevator. A middle-aged man entered the elevator and rode along with them just long enough to turn and tell them that I was going to be okay. Then the man got off the elevator, and they never saw him again!

"Dad, was that another Angel?" Sarah asked.

"I guess so. I've never seen him before, and I guess we'll never see him again. It's the third time we've gotten the message that Mom's going to be okay. We have to believe that. Whenever our hope flags, we need to remember these messages."

The daily surgeries were taking a toll on me, so much so that the doctors decided to switch to every other day. I had not eaten in days. The nausea, retching, and horrific unending pain had worn me down. The pain was always more severe at night, when everyone else was asleep. Sometimes a minute was more than I could handle. And then the next minute came and the next. I felt as if I had waged war on a thousand battlefields without ever leaving my hospital bed. Painful minutes turned into hours, hours into days, and days slowly became weeks.

My friend Heather moved into our home to take care of Adam and Sarah. She was single and had no ties to anyone. She knew both kids well, and they loved her and looked up to her as if she were their grown-up sister. They could talk to her about what scared them, about the next surgeries, about how much they missed having their mom wake them up for school. She knew where Adam was dropped off for the bus, and Sarah's middle school was just a minute from the elementary school where Heather and I worked. After school, Heather brought the kids to visit me.

Adam had an innate interest in the medical procedures. Sarah did not. She was terrified of anything medical. When she visited me, before she entered the room, I had someone drape me from neck to toes with a sheet so that she couldn't see anything. We couldn't talk about upcoming tests, surgeries, or other procedures in her presence. When the nurses attended me, she left the room.

One day my room was fairly crowded with visitors when Brooke came in to let everyone know she was going to change my dressings. Carole and Lindsay asked if they could stay, and Brooke didn't object. Sarah asked Eric, Lindsay's brother, if he'd go with her to the Atrium downstairs while my dressings were changed, and he said yes.

"Please stay together and come back in a few minutes," Rod said.

Eric had never been down to the Atrium, so Sarah showed him around the large space filled with stores and cafés. In the center was a beautiful fountain that provided ambient, relaxing sounds, surrounded by tables and chairs. A cathedral ceiling allowed visitors to look up for several floors. On one side, there were stairs that gracefully climbed from both sides to the second level. On that level was a large glass wall that allowed you to watch the visitors milling about. From the Atrium, you could also enter the Pediatric wing. A huge elephant made from colorful Legos stood more than a story high and marked the entrance.

With the hustle and bustle of people moving in all directions, instead of finding a seat, Sarah sat on the edge of the large fountain and Eric did the same. They talked for a bit. As Sarah looked around, she noticed a woman with long, dark hair standing on the second floor at the large glass wall watching her. Sarah stared back, then turned to Eric and said, "I want you to look up to the second floor where the wall of glass is and see if a lady with long, dark hair is staring at us."

He turned his body and looked up at the window. He saw the same woman. "Yep, she's definitely looking at us! Do you know her?"

"Nope."

Sarah looked up at the woman again, then watched in amazement as the lady pointed to her eye, then pointed to her heart, then pointed directly at Sarah.

Sarah said, "Did you see that?"

"No," he said. They both turned to find her again, but she had vanished.

"Eric, she gave me the "I love you" sign that only my mom and Adam and I know about. How did she know it and where did she go? If she would have walked in either direction, we would have seen her. But she just disappeared! I'm scared. Let's get out of here." They ran to the elevator and were relieved when the door opened immediately. They stepped inside and pressed seven.

"Eric?"

"What?"

"What if the doors open and she's standing there? What are we going to do?"

"Run!" was all he could get out as the doors opened. They ran all the way back to my room. They were both out of breath when they arrived. Sarah gasped as she tried to explain the visitor from the second floor, and the angelic message she had for Sarah.

"Don't be afraid," I said. "That was another Angel sent to give you a message of love. God shared our sign with an Angel so she could deliver it to you. You have no reason to be afraid."

Peace came over Sarah. Knowing that in time everything was going to be okay gave us all a strong feeling of hope. The Lord really was in charge.

CHAPTER 23

THE COMMUNITY CARES

John Mudry was the principal of our school. He was a wonderful leader and under his administration we were an Instructor A Plus School. He sat with Rod during that first, long night I was in surgery, and he visited often. Looking out for my best interests, he made an announcement at school that because of how injured I was, visitors were not permitted at the hospital. Instead, the teachers had their students make handwritten cards for me, which arrived by the hundreds. I was too sick to read the cards, but my family read every single one of them to me, then showed me the colorful pictures and taped the cards on every square inch of the walls. When they ran out of walls, they decorated the bed, then the ceiling.

A lovely woman I never met named Lorraine wrote me heartfelt and encouraging letters, which my family also read to me. She explained that she, too, had been in a bad accident—while walking in a large parking lot—and she also required many surgeries. She sent me at least one letter a month that first year. I felt isolated and alone much of the time. It meant so much to me to hear from someone who knew how I felt and what I was dealing with. Each time a letter arrived from Lorraine, I made sure someone read it to me before I dozed off again.

I received special blankets covered in children's handprints as well as a prayer blanket knitted in a soft yarn with a message that explained how prayers were said for me the entire time the blanket was being knitted. I was overwhelmed by this act of kindness. My tears flowed as I hugged the pale teal blanket to my face and chest. That blanket kept me warm, gave me peace, and went along with me into every surgery.

The school sent video recordings of the school children singing songs and performing skits for me as well as other recordings with special messages. A portable TV with a video player was wheeled into my room so I could watch them. Because of the pain, I could only watch small segments at a time. The highlight was the video showing the children planting a flower garden in front of the school in my honor. I wept for quite a while after I watched that tape. Parents told me that when they drove by the school and saw the beautiful flowers in bloom, they always thought of me. A plaque with my name on it is posted in the garden.

There were many other gifts and acts of kindness. I'm sure I've forgotten to include many of them. In the past I had more often been the giver of gifts like these than the receiver. People pleaser that I always have been, these gifts were sometimes difficult for me to accept. But what else could I do but accept them humbly and graciously?

✦ ✦ ✦

Mother's Day weekend was approaching. Rod asked me if I wanted anything special. I remember thinking, *I have at least forty bouquets of flowers in this room, so what more could I want?* We sent flowers to other patients, to the nurse's station, to the Church, and to shut-ins from the congregation. I certainly didn't need more flowers.

"I don't want anything this year," I said, feeling sorry for myself. *But I'd love to have my hair done. That might cheer me up.* "Unless you could get my hairdresser to come in. Michelle's phone number is at home in the silver address book."

"I'll see what I can do," he said.

By the next evening, I had forgotten all about my request as pain and nausea consumed me. That day I had undergone another debridement surgery, but this time after the procedure they placed a wound-vac on my leg. The wound-vac, also called vacuum-assisted closure, provides an airtight seal over the wound and gently applies suction. The suction reduces swelling, stimulates the growth of new tissue, and prevents infection. The suction also allows a superficial blood supply to be established along the wound's surface. In my case, I needed a greater blood supply to create the proper environment for a skin graft. As soon as the blood supply was established, according to Dr. Shin, he could begin skin graft surgery.

The next day Michelle and her daughter paid me a surprise visit with all her hairdressing supplies. I smiled from ear to ear in excitement. The nurses gave her a special tray to place in the bed under my head, to divert the rinse water into a trash can on the floor. I really wasn't feeling well, but when I saw my reflection in the mirror, I knew I needed to do something about that scraggly mess.

Michelle took her time. She applied the hair color first, and I drifted in and out of sleep while the dye set. Afterwards she washed my hair so thoroughly and deeply that it had the effect of a deep massage. I wasn't quite sure how she'd cut my hair while I was lying in bed, but she was a miracle worker. Nothing was an obstacle for her that day, and she was pleasant and funny as well. God, did I need that diversion. She told me she'd be back every three weeks. She was an angel of a different kind, but an angel nonetheless.

On the Friday evening of Mother's Day weekend, I was surprised when one of my best friends, Kelly, walked into the room with suitcase in hand. She was the one who had driven me to the hospital the day Adam was born. We had graduated from the same nursing program and worked in critical care together at two different hospitals. The kids lovingly call her Aunt Kelly, and I call her my sister, since I was never blessed with a biological sister. And there she was, standing before me. All I could do was cry. It was obvious to both of us that the road ahead of me would be rocky, with many bumps and detours along the way. But when I saw her and the loving way she looked at me, I knew I'd never have to walk that path alone.

After all the tears and greetings, Kelly put her suitcase down and looked at Rod as she spoke. "I'm your weekend respite care. I've come to spend Mother's Day weekend with my best friend. So why don't you and the kids go down to Wildwood for the weekend and enjoy the beach? It's supposed to be a beautiful weekend."

"You'll miss Mother's Day with Marlee!" Rod protested. Marlee is Kelly's daughter.

"Marlee understands. I'm going to celebrate this year with Kim. I've brought plenty of things to do. To pamper her I've brought along lotions for back rubs and massages to her arms and legs. I brought nail polish. I'll give her a mani-pedi. I've got magazines and Mad Libs. So go home, pack your bags, and head to the Shore."

Rod turned to me. "Should we Kim?"

"I think it's a great idea," I smiled and nodded. "You guys need a break. The kids will be so excited. Besides, you're leaving me with the best critical care nurse I know."

After our good-byes and I love yous, Rod left. I teared up when I said to Kelly, "Thank you for coming, especially this weekend. It's so good to see you. I love you, my sister!"

"I love you, too. Rod didn't get a chance to call me until two days after the accident. I got here as soon as I could take a few days off." She took my hand and held it tightly with both of hers. "How's your pain level?"

"Awful. Somedays I don't know how I'm going to get through another minute."

"What are they giving you?'

"A Dilaudid drip."

"If I push this button, will you get more?"

"Yes. It's programmed for every ten minutes."

"I haven't seen you press the button since I got here, so I'm going to press it so you'll get a little more."

I felt a weird sensation as the dose entered my bloodstream. I closed my eyes and fell into a kind of drugged half-sleep.

Kelly told me about this next part later.

While I was out of it, she took the elevator to the first floor so she could go outside to call her husband, Bob. In the hustle and bustle orbiting the large medical center, she punched in the numbers for her husband. When he answered, she tried to speak, but broke down sobbing instead.

"Kell?"

"Umm hum," she said, sobbing.

"Is it that bad?"

"YES!" was all she managed to get out. There was a period of silence before she spoke again. "I feel so helpless. My heart just aches for her. I've never seen legs so bad. I can't imagine what she went through and what she still has to go through. I'm so glad I came. Are you and Marlee okay?"

"We're fine," he said. "You can have her on Father's Day."

"I made Rod and the kids go to Wildwood for the weekend. I'm going to stay in her room."

"That's good. Give Kim my love."

Kelly slipped quietly back into the room so she wouldn't disturb me. Only a small amount of light from the city below crept through the wall of windows. Kelly padded to my bedside and saw my eyes open. "Are you having pain again?"

All I could do was nod, hoping that, like Rod, Kelly would understand that sometimes the pain was too intense for me to talk. Every morning I prayed for the day to end, but when nighttime arrived, I prayed for the morning. I couldn't win. Although my friends and family could do a great deal for me—arranging my blankets, reading cards and letters, chatting to help pass the time—no one could suffer with me, no one could take the pain away. That I could only do alone even in a room full of visitors. At the same time, I always knew the Lord was with me and that he had much bigger things in mind. Sometimes I thought He was all that kept me going.

"I'll push your button again," Kelly said. "Are you cold? Is that why you're shaking?"

I shook my head. The trembling intensified.

"If this doesn't help, I'll talk to the nurse to see what else we can do. I promise, you won't suffer on my watch!"

I felt the same weird jolt from the medication, but this time the stabbing bone pain was intensified by involuntary muscle spasms, as if the muscles were being ripped from my bones. I didn't know what to do. Should I sit up? Should I lower my head? I didn't know. Maybe if I rubbed my legs or held onto them tightly. I desperately looked to Kelly for the answers without saying a word.

Good friend that she is, she got it. "It's okay, don't try to talk. I'm going to find your nurse and get you something else for pain." She left the room.

Just when I thought they would never return, they did. They gave me more medicine with an IV push. I felt the heavy sedative's effects immediately and watched the room twirl in odd patterns until I drifted off.

Kelly stayed awake as long as she could to press the Dilaudid button at the precise intervals permitted. When she finally got into bed, she begged God to heal me quickly and relieve my pain.

Her sleep, like mine, was tormented with nightmares. She woke to my screams of terror in the middle of the night. When she appeared at my bedside in the dimly lit room, I didn't know who she was.

"Are you okay?" She touched me on the shoulder, afraid to do more.

Ah, Kelly, I said to myself when I recognized her voice. *Oh, thank God. It was just a nightmare, another nightmare.* "Nightmares wake me up every night," I said aloud. "They're always different, but they come with the same intense terror until I wake myself screaming. Then I'm too afraid to fall back to sleep. But sleep is the only thing that gives me any relief, no matter how small. I ask the doctors again and again. When will this be over? When will I get back to normal? They never answer me, but I keep asking. I keep on asking."

"How about a back rub? That might relax you. And I can rub lotion on your arms and hands too. Your skin is so dry."

"That sounds wonderful!"

She retrieved her lotions from her night bag. I was only able to roll slightly due to the traction and wound-vac. She reached in behind me, and with the softest of strokes, she applied the cool lotion. I sighed with pleasure. Since the accident, touch had brought only pain, and this was heavenly. Her smooth, gentle hands and the aroma of lavender soothed me into deep relaxed breaths. Nothing I had experienced in the previous two weeks had felt this wonderful. When she finished my back, she moved to my arms and hands. This also felt wonderful, but all too soon, she had to stop.

"Can you go back to sleep?" she asked while she replaced the caps on the lotions. "Or should I find us a cup of hot tea?"

"Tea please," I said, surprised that that sounded good to me.

She disappeared into the hallway. She returned holding two paper cups with the teabag tag hanging off the lip. "How's English Breakfast?"

"Perfect," I said, and it was. Though I couldn't finish it, whatever I was able to drink had never tasted so good.

The day progressed from that point, filled with tears and laughter and more tears. We filled in the blanks of several Mad Lib Books, polished my fingernails and toenails, and talked. Nothing too deep. Mostly catching up and practical stuff about my condition. What I desperately wanted to talk about with someone, though, was how I was afraid I was losing my mind, that the pain was breaking me, literally driving me crazy. How could I bring that up with Kelly or anyone else? Everyone was already too stressed with the day-to-day challenges and my constant pain. I couldn't burden them with this as well. So I kept it to myself, although it scared me to my soul. What if I never came back from this, physically *or* mentally?

This new paranoia manifested itself in strange ways. When Kelly wanted to turn on the TV to the morning news, I made up an excuse to watch another channel when, in fact, I was simply too frightened to hear the news. It was all so tragic and traumatic.

On Saturday, Rod and the kids called. I assured them I was doing fine, that Kelly was a perfect caregiver and advocate in their absence. They planned to return the next day, so I told them to enjoy the beach.

And that was no lie. Kelly was the perfect caregiver. Before the pain ever got out of control, she made sure I pushed the magic button—or she pushed it herself. As a result, I dozed off and on throughout the day, jolted awake by bad dreams and pain as the day passed into yet another long night filled with even more pain and torment. Minutes were hours, hours were days, and days, well, days became an eternity of agony with no relief in sight. I begged God for relief, but it never came. I was exhausted, but I couldn't get any rest. Truly, if this wasn't hell on earth, I didn't know what was. Kelly came to my bedside when she saw my pain and did whatever she could to help or distract me. I was grateful for these small mercies, but I was profoundly alone in my suffering.

By Sunday afternoon, the kids and Rod returned with arms full of food for everyone. Some days the room seemed more like a fast-food restaurant. At least that day, the smells didn't induce instant nausea and retching.

Kelly stayed for a few more hours, but she had a four-hour drive ahead of her, and we finally had to say our sad goodbyes. Though she did her best to hide her feelings behind her nurse's strength, her expression was a heartbreaking mixture of compassion, hope, despair, and fear, as if she would have done anything to take that pain away from me, the pain in the moment as well as the pain to come. She was too much the nurse to pretend she didn't know what I was facing. All she could do for me was pray, pray like she never had before, and

I knew she would, as she had done that whole weekend. Kelly's faith, like mine, had developed at a very young age. We were both blessed with devout mothers who passed their faith onto us. I believe that the most important thing we can do is to pray for others. Prayer is not something we can do only for ourselves. It is our chance to break the bread and to drink the wine in communion with our fellow men and women, to offer everyone God's comfort and compassion.

✦ ✦ ✦

After that brief respite from surgery, the medical team reminded me that we had to do skin grafts to close the gaping wound on the back of my left leg. The wound-vac had done its job improving the circulation to the surface of the remaining calf muscle. They planned to use tissue from my upper thighs. Surgery would be in the morning. Thanks for the warning!

There had been another medical issue nagging me, and in a moment of relative clarity, I finally addressed it with Dr. Yue. I asked him, with all the surgeries I was going through, whether I needed an internal filter to prevent blood clots and fat emboli from traveling to my heart or brain, causing a heart attack or stroke. Dr. Yue acknowledged that they had forgotten all about that. Later that afternoon, I was taken to the Interventional Radiology Department, where a greenfield filter was inserted into my Inferior Vena Cava through the right jugular vein in my neck. They followed up with an x-ray to make sure it was properly in place. My nursing background may have saved my life, and not for the first or last time.

CHAPTER 24

DISAPPOINTMENT PREVAILS

The skin graft surgery was scheduled early in the morning. Dr. Shin's residents woke me up to describe the surgery. They planned to harvest the skin from my left thigh to place on the posterior left calf where the muscle had been lost.

I finished my bed bath just before the transport team arrived. I said goodbye to Rod as they wheeled my bed into the hallway. Anxiety hit me the second the transport team pushed me into the hallway. I hadn't been able to drink water in the previous eight hours and my mouth was so dry I could barely swallow. I was breathing fast, practically hyperventilating, but I felt like I wasn't getting enough air in my lungs. My heart raced as I scanned the hall ahead of me. *Why am I so afraid?* Every muscle seemed tight, ready to spasm. I closed my eyes and told myself that I was almost there! I could smell that we were getting closer, literally. Once I heard the whoosh of the OR doors, I knew we made it. I was safe once again.

A few hours later, I woke in the recovery room with my left thigh on fire. I took a peek under the covers. A thin, yellow, Vaseline impregnated piece of medicated gauze covered a large area of the thigh.

I couldn't sleep well that night because of the intense burning. Finally, in the wee hours of the morning, exhaustion took over, and I fell into sleep—until the residents snapped on the overhead lights what seemed like minutes later.

"Time to remove your bandages, Mrs. Shipe," said one of the residents as they approached my bed. I squinted as they lowered the sheets. They put waterproof pads on the bed and cracked open a bottle of sterile saline.

"This is going to feel cold," the male resident said as he poured the saline over my thigh dressing. Then without warning, he tore the dressing from my thigh. I wailed in pain. "We're going to leave the dressings off," he explained. "But we aren't going to remove the dressing at the grafting site until six days post-op."

"Next time give me the bottle of saline, and I'll remove my own damn dressing," I said.

They turned in unison and walked out. I shook my head. *Did they practice that in the breakroom?* The wound on my thigh wept a pale-yellow fluid, which stuck to my top sheet. Every time I moved, the sheet tore away from the wound, and the site burned all over again.

Finally, it was day six. Dr. Shin and his residents arrived early. With precision, Dr. Shin slowly and steadily removed the dressing from the graft site. When he finished, the residents looked at him, first in confusion, then with disappointment.

"The skin graft didn't take. We have to go back to the OR to debride the site before we try again," Dr. Shin announced in his professionally flat voice.

This was the first attempt at a skin graft, but many more were required. The next four were successful, but the three procedures on the anterior part of my leg after that failed. The anterior site required a muscle flap and artery transfer before it could be successfully closed.

Dr. Shin and one of his colleagues performed the twelve-hour surgery to transfer a muscle and artery from my left forearm to my left leg. One morning after that surgery, Dr. Shin's residents entered my room and told me they were instructed to debride an area on my left leg. They planned to do it right there, at my bedside!

"Oh no, no no," I said. "No, no, no. I always go to the operating room for debridement under anesthesia."

"Don't worry. You won't feel anything when we cut," one of the residents said. "It's dead tissue."

"If you say so," I said, not really convinced.

Another resident opened the sterile pack of instruments, gloves, and drapes, and placed them in position. Then he snapped on a pair of sterile gloves and picked up the scalpel and started to carve the dead tissue away.

"Yow," I screeched. "STOP! I can feel every cut. Do NOT touch me again until I'm under anesthesia!"

"Dr. Shin told us to do this today," he argued. Then he turned to another member of the crew. "Page anesthesia now!"

Within a few minutes an anesthesiologist joined us in the room carrying several syringes. The residents explained their dilemma. Then the doctor walked over to me and said he was going to put me under.

"But we're going to the OR," I said.

"No, I'll do it right here in your room." He located my IV and started to push the medicine through the line. As a nurse—and a patient—I was concerned. I wasn't on a heart monitor, no one had checked my blood pressure, and I wasn't getting any oxygen. Before I could object, I lost consciousness.

I don't know how long I was unconscious. I came to to the sound of my nurse tearing the residents and anesthesiologist a new one. "Who told you you could put my patient under anesthesia? Are you all crazy? She wasn't being monitored. No one even told me you were going to do this here. It's an orthopedic unit for crying out loud. I'm notifying the nursing supervisor. NEVER do that again!" She paged the nursing supervisor, then walked out of the room to talk in private. Meanwhile, the two residents and the anesthesiologist slunk away.

"Are you okay?" Brooke asked when she reentered the room.

"Yeah, just nauseated from the anesthesia."

The rest of the day was quiet, though interrupted by waves of severe pain and nausea. I don't know if the residents or the anesthesiologist were reprimanded for attempting to perform surgery in the room, but I certainly didn't see them or Dr. Shin that day.

By evening, my pain had gotten so intense that even the strongest of narcotics did little to stop the spasms in my lower legs. I tried different positions, and when that did little to help, I sobbed, rocking my body from side to side. I asked Rod, "Why is my pain always worse at night?" For Rod it was a rhetorical question, but the doctors I asked had no explanation either.

In agony, I prayed out loud, begging God to let me die. I'm sure that upset Rod, but I had had it. Death seemed to be the best solution to all my misery.

I don't know how to describe such unimaginable pain, but I'll try. This was what went through my mind when I was in that kind of pain:

Sit up, lie down. Move, don't move. Take medicine, don't take medicine. Flush the pills down the toilet so I won't get addicted. The nausea, vomiting, and dry heaves come no matter what. Eat, don't eat. Drink water, drink nothing. The sweating, chills, tremors, and restlessness come no matter what. Relax, find a diversion, do nothing. Talk, don't talk, grind your teeth. The contortions and screaming and hallucinations come no matter what. Pray, don't pray, ask others to pray. Watch TV, turn off the TV. Read a magazine, close the magazine. Turn in bed, don't turn in bed. Cry, don't cry. Smile, don't smile. Breathe slowly and deeply. Breathe rapidly and shallowly. The loneliness, frustration, and desperation come no matter what, even when surrounded by loved ones because surely they won't stand by me forever in this condition.

So, I pretend. Pretend that everything's fine, that I feel no pain, that I don't daily think of ending it all. But the pain comes at night, the pain comes in the day. I can't think straight. I can't remember simple things. I can't remember what I don't remember. What am I going to do if the pain never goes away? I'll just end it all. That's the ticket. No, I can't do that to my family.

And when the pain mercifully subsides, however briefly, I brace myself because I know it's coming back. It's going to start all over again, an endless cycle of pain and more pain. If hell is the endless repetition of punishment, then this is hell indeed. I call it the face of pain. Anyone who has ever had pain can relate. It is all-consuming, and you feel very much alone because you are in so much pain no one else can possibly understand.

The crazy thing about pain of this magnitude is that there's only a fairly narrow window in which the medication works, a window that's difficult to predict. If you put off taking the meds, you risk missing that window, and the pain simply gets out of control—it literally becomes too much. When that happens, even if you take the medicine, it often doesn't help.

Because I hated to use the pain medicine, I often missed the window, and not only did I have to deal with the pain for a lot longer than I should have, I also had to face an angry family who didn't understand why I just didn't take the damn meds when (as they saw it) I was supposed to! They didn't understand how afraid I was of getting addicted, that this was my way of proving to myself that I wasn't addicted. It was difficult to be accountable to my beliefs and family at the same time!

That night, Rod called in the nurse to get the doctor to find something that worked. Within a short amount of time, they administered additional IV painkiller, and I finally drifted off, tormented by the nightmares I had whenever I fell asleep. I'd wake up in a panic, then thank God when I realized the dreams weren't real.

In the early hours of the night, I woke up with an intense itch on the bottom of my left foot. Both of my legs were suspended in mid-air in traction, and I had cobalt blue metal fixators on both lower legs, which prevented me from reaching my foot. The room was pitch black and I could hear Rod snoring quietly on the cot at the bottom of my bed. *It's not fair to wake him in the middle of the night because my foot itches*, I thought to myself.

I remembered that a single metal piece extended from the back of my right foot about three inches beyond the fixator. If I maneuvered properly, I could use it to scratch the itch on the bottom of my left foot. I squinted, trying to focus my vision in a dark room, but I couldn't see a thing. I raised my right leg and turned it outward, then brought it toward my left foot. But I miscalculated, and instead of hitting the itch, I tangled the fixators. I tried to move the fixators apart, but I couldn't disentangle them. Nothing else I tried worked either. *What am I going to do?*

The only thing I could do was wake up Rod. I quietly called his name, then I called it a little louder. He bounced off the cot and quickly walked to the head of my bed.

"Are you okay? What's going on?" He switched on the light. We both turned our eyes from the sudden glare.

"My fixators got tangled!"

"What the Hell are you doing?" he yelled, still half asleep. "Are you hallucinating? I'm getting the nurse. I can't untangle those things!" Then he stomped off to find the nurse. After Rod returned with the nurse, it took her five minutes to free the legs. It was like one of those logic puzzles you can buy at a game store. I decided not to mention that all this had happened because I was trying to scratch an itch on the bottom of my foot.

The next day, Rod retold that story many times, embellishing it each time. By the end of the week, it was nothing like what had actually happened. That's when I told him the truth. That I was just trying to scratch an itch. He was surprised to learn I hadn't been hallucinating! Of course, he embellished that story, too. He had me hanging in the air by my fixators virtually upside down.

CHAPTER 25

A BRIEF HOMECOMING

Twenty-four hours were more than I could handle most days. The intense pain was unbearable. Dilaudid worked better than morphine, and I could administer it myself with that magic button. Unfortunately, due to the extreme nausea and vomiting, I couldn't really eat, and I was losing too much weight. To give my poor body a break, the medical team tried to extend the time between surgeries.

Mentally, however, I got no breaks. Flashbacks of the accident terrorized me day and night. I'd be minding my own business—talking to Rod or a nurse or just closing my eyes against the harsh hospital lights, and all of a sudden, I'd see a vivid vision of myself, as vivid and as real as the nurse giving me a sponge bath, with dangling, twisted legs that were ready to fall off. My heart raced, and I broke out in a dripping sweat that required a frequent change in linens. Nighttime was no better. If I could actually manage to fall asleep, the night terrors jolted me awake. I couldn't get any rest. Along with the nurses' visits and dressing changes, early dawn doctor visits, physical therapy, morning surgeries, pain and vomiting, I was worn out! *Was I losing my mind?*

I thought maybe I should mention it to Brooke, the nurse, when Rod and the kids were gone, as embarrassing as it might be. Why was I so afraid? I wasn't the kind to scare easily. I had been a critical care nurse. I was always the strong one. But I was at the end of my rope. Even trips to the operating room freaked me out.

When I was finally alone, I pushed the call button.

I told the aide who answered that I wanted to talk to my nurse. Within a few minutes, Brooke came into my room. "What's up?" she said in her professionally cheerful voice. "What do you need?"

Brooke looked at me expectantly, but I didn't know how to begin.

Brooke touched my arm and said, "It's okay. You can tell me anything."

Then I launched into it. "I waited until no one was here to tell you this. I feel like I'm losing my mind, that I'm going crazy. I'm scared of everything. I can't turn off my brain. Everything makes me jump. I imagine crashing into the walls in the hallway, and the intense pain I'd feel if I did. I imagine falling off the bed. I imagine someone grabbing my fixators and pulling my legs off. And that's just the fake stuff. I remember in vivid flashbacks how my legs looked just after the accident, like they were hanging by a thread. I can't sleep, I can't rest, I'm exhausted. I'm going a little bit nuts here."

"Oh, Kim," she said, taking me by the hand. "Of course you feel that way. You're dealing with so much right now, with the accident, the surgeries, the pain, the helplessness. Your world is spinning out of control. Of course you feel off. Way off. You're not losing your mind— at least not permanently!" She smiled, and I couldn't help but smile back. Then she turned serious again. "I'll ask our psychiatric nurse to drop by."

Help at last, I thought.

In late afternoon, Nancy arrived. With four simple letters, she cleared up the mystery. "P-T-S-D," she said. "With that kind of accident, you likely have PTSD."

Ah, yes, PTSD, I thought. I should have known. I'd had it before—when I was raped as a teenager. But it had felt different then. I supposed that PTSD feels different each time you experience it.

Now that I could put a name to how I was feeling, I felt instant relief. I wasn't over it, not by a longshot, but I knew it was normal, expected after such a traumatic accident. I wasn't losing my mind, not exactly. Nancy emphasized the importance of staying in the moment, of not letting my mind wander into the horrors of the past or to over-anticipate future dangers. One way to do that, she explained, was to keep a calendar nearby. She noticed I didn't have one. After she left, she returned an hour later and taped a handmade calendar to the wall. "There you go," she said, pointing to one of the squares. "That's today. Try not to think about anything else but that little square." Then she said she'd see me the next day. It was nice to have someone to talk to besides Brooke and Rod.

Not that Rod wasn't a great support. He had taken a leave of absence from Truelove and McClean, in Waterbury, Connecticut, where he was the Global Vice President of the commercial department. He very rarely left my side, and was at my beck and call to rearrange pillows or get me ice water or applesauce and all of that. He was my husband, and he wanted to fix things for me. He wanted me to feel better. He got it into his head that what I needed was to get home, that if I got home, my spirits would lift, that things would be on the way back to normal. The first couple of times he asked about my going home, Dr. Yue said, "Absolutely not." That didn't stop Rod, though. He asked just about every day.

I wasn't so sure about going home. I felt safe in the hospital, with all the life-saving equipment and help five seconds away with the call button. Rod was much more excited by the prospect than I was. I trusted that Dr. Yue wouldn't let me leave until I was ready.

Weeks passed. Rod pleaded with the doctors daily, and one morning, to the surprise of us all, Dr Yue said, "Yes," but that Rod would have to meet with a social worker to order the equipment I'd need at home.

In the meantime, Rod's dad, who I called Pop, arrived from Florida to help out for a few weeks while I was home. The support of family was one thing that kept me going. He was more than a father-in-law. I loved him very much.

The ambulance was arranged for the end of the week.

The closer we got to the day of departure, the more I fretted. I really, really, really didn't want to leave the safety of the hospital. All I saw were potential booby traps ahead—what if it hurt too much to travel, what if I reinjured myself, what if nobody at home knew how to work the equipment? It was overwhelming! These and other anxieties ricocheted around my brain, making my heart race and my gut queasy. Nightmares about going home replaced the nightmares about the accident. Finally, I said something to Rod. "Why do I have to go home again? I feel safe here!"

"You're going to feel so much better at home for a few days. Besides, it's happening. Everything's being delivered today. I have to head home this afternoon to wait for the medical supplier."

"I hate it when you aren't here."

"We'll only be apart for a few hours. You can take a nap before you leave."

I almost cried when Rod left the room. I didn't want to be alone, and I didn't want to go home either. Waves of doubt crashed into me. *What if we're in an accident on the way home? I don't even know the ambulance driver. What's his safety record? Has he gotten any tickets? Is he having a good day? Will he be well-rested and alert?* I couldn't help thinking like this. Shortly after I drifted into sleep, I woke up to tortured dreams. I tried to focus on the positive. I was looking forward to seeing our dog, Madison. Several weeks earlier, Rod had surprised me by bringing her to the hospital for a visit. He had given her some sedation as recommended by the vet, but she was so drugged up that after briefly kissing my hands, she fell asleep on Rod's cot.

The only other time Rod had left me was for the weekend he had to coach Sarah's AAU team at a tournament in New York state. That, too, panicked me. My principal, John Mudry, had visited me just before that weekend while I was in the midst of a delirious and pain-filled day. I begged him to find someone to sleep with me for the weekend. He kept a straight face and said he would take care of that. Then he placed a cool washcloth onto my forehead and stroked my hair as I drifted back into a narcotics-induced sleep. He arranged for Heather, my running partner, to take Adam to a friend's house for the weekend so she could stay at the hospital with me. On John's next visit, we laughed at how I had phrased my request—that I needed someone to sleep with me.

All that day the nurses, doctors, and aides stopped in to say good-bye. I was sad and scared. I watched the clock on the wall. My stomach started to hurt, and my heart raced the closer the clock got to the mag-ical hour. *This is stupid. Why, why do I have to do this?*

Suddenly two strong men entered my room with their litter. They could have been football players.

"Are you Kim Shipe?"

I thought about denying it, but they probably had paperwork to prove me wrong. "Yes, I am."

"Well, we're here to take you home," they said cheerfully, as if that was a good thing.

How could I explain to them that it was the last thing I wanted to do just then! "Okay," I rasped, my throat closing up in anxiety. Several nurses came into the room to assist with my transfer from the bed to the litter. My thoughts raced, I sweated buckets, my heart pounded, my eyes filled with tears.

"You're going to be fine," Brooke said as the attendants pushed me—none too carefully!—towards the elevator. As we approached the nursing station, I heard the good-bye shouts, but all I could muster in response was a half wave. *This is all PTSD*, I told myself. *Don't be afraid. The Lord is with me. He will protect me. Right Lord? You're going to protect me?* I was surfing the knife edge of emotions.

When the double doors opened to the ambulance bay, I took in the sounds of birds chirping and traffic moving. The warmth of the sun on my face felt good. I remembered running in the cool of the mornings. When the sun came out, everything felt brand new. Would I ever feel that again? I took a slow deep breath. They loaded me into the ambulance, slammed the doors behind me, and the thrill ride began.

Oh God, why do they put windows in the back of ambulances? That car is tailgating. Don't they know this is an ambulance? Back off, Jack. Oh dear, he almost rear-ended us. Did you guys even take driver's ed?

And so on, a running inner commentary of anxiety. It's no wonder my blood pressure went sky high. When we hit a bump, the spasms hit, and the pain was awful, even though they had given me a dose of morphine for the ride.

In my head I was measuring the distance to the house—two miles, one mile, half a mile, three driveways. I helped steer the ambulance by gripping the stretcher's handrails and weaving into the turns. It was only when I heard the beep-beep-beep of the ambulance backing down our slightly graded driveway that I unclenched my fists.

When the double doors opened, I saw the kids holding balloons and flowers to welcome me home, along with Rod, Heather, and Pop, who had Madison by the collar. Everyone hollered, "Welcome home!" in unison. I smiled. Madison was straining to get away from Pop. Pop let her come close enough to sniff me. Madison's excitement let me know I was truly home. I knew she'd be sleeping close to me that night.

CHAPTER 26

RESPITE CUT SHORT

A s soon as the paramedics got me into bed, I felt a peace come over me, and I instantly knew that Rod had been right, being home was a good idea, even if it would be short lived.

The worries I had about the home equipment were quickly dispelled. I had the most comfortable air pressure mattress that constantly readjusted as I moved. I had lost so much weight that every boney prominence needed to be protected from breakdown. They installed a trapeze bar, so I could hoist myself up in the bed. I had oxygen tanks hidden at the head of the bed. I had a nice wheelchair and even a transfer board to assist me in getting from the bed to the wheelchair. At the hospital, they had just recently started to get me out of bed and into a wheelchair with both of my legs elevated straight in front of me.

I still couldn't use a bathroom on my own, so that meant a bedpan. They had just removed the foley catheter and told me that due to the length of time it was in, I'd have to be patient until I got full bladder control back. Boy were they right! One small laugh, and the dam ruptured!

When I was settled in, Pop asked Rod to meet him in the dining room where I was quietly resting in bed.

Pop said, "I want you and the kids to go to Wildwood. I'll take care of Kim for the weekend. You haven't taken a break in weeks, and you're so thin! The kids need a break too. Kim is in good hands with me. You know that. Now go and pack. I'm not taking, *no* for an answer!"

"Kim are you okay with this?" Rod said to me.

"Yes, Pop knows how to take care of people. Look at how long he cared for Francis." Francis was Pop's mother-in-law, who had passed away after a long illness.

I did feel sad about them leaving me as soon as I got home, but Rod had brightened at the idea, and I couldn't say no. I knew Pop would be good company. He understood PTSD, having retired as a full-bird Colonel many years after serving in the U.S. Air Force. He had flown over four hundred missions in Vietnam.

Once they realized I was okay with the plan, the kids were excited too.

"Okay, let's get packed," Rod called out, and all three of them headed to their rooms.

That's when it dawned on me. Pop would have to help with the bedpans and washing up! Another wave of anxiety hit me, and I blushed. *How will we both handle that?* I wondered. *It's not like I can hold it for two days.*

"Pop ...?"

"Yes?"

"I just realized that you'll be handling the bedpan while I pull myself up on the trapeze. That's a little—mortifying. You'll see everything, you know what I mean?"

"I'm fine with that if you are. Don't give it another thought."

"Okay, Pop," I said, still not entirely sure I was okay with it. "I love you so much. You're my favorite father-in-law!" Then we both laughed at the old joke.

"I got your favorite for dinner tomorrow. A filet mignon on the grill. Tonight, we'll just have hamburgers and corn on the cob."

"That sounds delicious, thank you. I just hope I have an appetite."

I dozed off until Rod and the kids woke me to say goodbye. I kissed everyone and told them to have fun and be safe. Then I returned to a sleep of deep exhaustion.

Pop woke me several hours later and handed me a plate holding an extremely rare hamburger dripping its juices from the bun, lima beans, and an ear of white sweet corn, already buttered and salted. "Boy, Pop, you're setting a high bar here. And you remembered the Lima beans. Thank you. I love you."

I gave it my all because everything looked and smelled so delicious after months of hospital food. I started with the burger since I knew how badly I needed protein. But my shrunken stomach filled up quickly. After several small bites of everything, I was full. Pop agreed to save it all for another meal.

Soon after dinner, Pop gave me a warm, soapy wash cloth along with toothpaste and a toothbrush. He also unwrapped the plastic bed-pan and brought it in for me to use. I was a little embarrassed, but Pop didn't make me feel uncomfortable in the least. "I'm going to give you a bell for the night. If you need me, I want you to ring it until I wake up, okay?"

"Sure, but I'm so tired. I'll be able to sleep all night. Just leave my pain medicine here and something to drink."

I fell asleep quickly. The next time I woke and looked around, it seemed like the entire first floor was dark and quiet, a welcome contrast to the noisy, bright hospital. Pop must have been sound asleep upstairs. The pain had grown, so I washed down a Dilaudid, thinking about Rod and the kids, hoping they had arrived safely. The pain slowly subsided, and I drifted back to sleep.

I woke in the morning to the sun peeking in the front windows and the aroma of coffee. It smelled wonderful. It smelled like home.

I could hear Pop in the kitchen, so I hollered, "Good morning, Pop."

"Good morning my favorite daughter-in-law!" I laughed as he walked into the dining room. "Are you ready for breakfast? The visiting nurse will be here around ten."

"Sure, I'm actually hungry this morning. What are you making?"

"How does scrambled eggs and bacon sound?"

"Amazing!"

Pop returned with breakfast in a few minutes, a single scrambled egg and three slices of bacon with fresh pineapple.

After a few bites, I said, "Pop I've never tasted eggs this good. So light and fluffy. And the perfect amount of salt."

"Want to know the trick?"

"I'd love to."

"It was my mom's secret. She always added a little water before she beat the eggs. That's why they get so fluffy."

"I'm going to steal that from now on!"

After breakfast and a bed bath, the visiting nurse arrived to change the sterile dressings on my legs. The physical therapist also stopped by to initiate therapy. Afterwards I drifted into a deep and restful nap that lasted hours until the pain brought me back to reality. Pop gave me pills for the pain and pills for the nausea. When both subsided, I ate a few small bites of a grilled cheese sandwich and a spoonful or two of tomato bisque. Then I fell asleep again.

This time when I woke up, Pop let me get oriented, then said, "I'm going to help you into your wheelchair so I can take you out on the back porch. It's such a beautiful day with a gentle breeze. I'm sure you'd like to be outside."

"No, you can't do that. How will you get me down the step? And the door's so narrow I'm not sure the wheelchair will fit."

"I've already measured the door frame, and the wheelchair *will* fit. You don't have to be afraid. I'll back you out the door. You'll be fine."

I was afraid—afraid of more pain, afraid of reinjuring myself. But I had to trust my caregivers. I was at their mercy. "Okay, we can try, but just so you know, I'm pretty nervous."

"You're going to be fine. I'll tell you everything I'm going to do before I do it."

By then I knew the drill. I lined up the transfer board with the side of the wheelchair as soon as Pop removed the side panel on the chair.

Ever so slowly I scooted across the board while Pop helped me by lifting my legs and placing them on the pillow across the leg rests.

Even simple transfers like this took a lot out of me, requiring strength, tenacity, and endurance I wasn't sure I had. Confined to a hospital bed for two full months, I had lost much of my muscle mass. When I looked into a mirror, all I saw were sunken eyes with dark circles underneath, as well as sucked in cheeks and sharp cheekbones that made me look one hundred years old. I looked awful, very sickly.

I grew short of breath as I maneuvered into the chair, and I was close to weeping with frustration. On April 30, the day before the accident, I had gone on a five-mile run with Heather without stopping. Now I couldn't even get myself into a chair two feet away.

But with Pop's help, I slid into the chair, and though I couldn't say I was comfortable, I was able to sit up, more or less, my hardware-encased legs sticking straight out on the leg rests. Pop slowly pushed me into the kitchen with Madison on my tail. She hadn't left my side since I came home. As I had been at the hospital and in the ambulance, I was hyperfocused on every potential hazard before us.

We moved carefully through the kitchen. Pop paused to nudge the table out of our way. At the porch door, he said, "I'm going to lift you over the threshold and then down the step onto the porch."

Then with surprising strength for a man his age, he lifted the back of my wheelchair to turn me into the correct alignment to get through the doorway.

"I'll keep my arms in," I said.

It was as if we had practiced a million times, and just like that, I was on the porch.

I tipped my head backwards with my eyes closed, allowing the sun to fall on my face, while the gentle summer breeze tousled my hair. Pop was right. It felt amazing to be back outside, listening to the birds chirping from the woods a hundred feet away. I opened my eyes to take it all in. Everything looked so beautiful. The flowers around the deck were in full bloom, and the burst of brilliant yellows, oranges, and pinks were spectacular up close. The subtlest of floral scents wafted my way like an expensive perfume. It was as pure as Heaven. I was glad to be alive, a feeling I seldom had had since the accident.

"Thanks for bringing me out, Pop. I'm happy we pushed through my fears!"

"I know how much you enjoy nature. I thought this might give you a new outlook. I'm going to leave you and Madison here while I make dinner."

For the next thirty or forty minutes, Madison and I were totally content, engrossed in the outdoors and at peace with one another. She looked like a grey ghost with her crisply colored eyes, golden-brown in the sunlight. She nudged me with her wet nose to pet her, and I did, running my fingers through the silky fur on her long floppy ears. She held herself tall and proud as she sat next to me. Did she miss our runs as much as I did? When I first arrived, she had sniffed at the still open wounds on my legs. I wondered what the scents meant to her. Did she understand the severity of my injuries? I thought she must have. That's why she stayed so close. My mind was always going a mile a minute those days. So many questions. So few answers.

Pop opened the door to announce dinner.

"Come along girl," he said to Madison, then let her inside. "Let's get you out of the way." After she was inside, he returned. "I'm going to bump you up over the threshold forward this time," he said releasing both brakes. He did exactly what he said he was going to do, and this time I wasn't afraid at all.

Dinner was excellent. I remained out of bed in my wheelchair until I could no longer keep my eyes open. We watched some TV, talked a bit, and spoke with Rod and the kids.

Finally I said, "I think the fresh air tired me out. I'm ready for bed."

I couldn't believe how tired I was. I figured I wouldn't have any trouble sleeping that night.

Pop brought me my bathroom kit, and I brushed my teeth and washed my face with warm water and a complexion bar. I turned to Madison and said, "Madison, are you ready for bed?" She slowly lifted her head, looking at me with bloodshot, droopy eyes as if to say, *Hell yes, I'm ready for bed!* As we got ready to make the transfer from the wheelchair to the bed, Madison flopped down on the floor to a moan of pure exhaustion.

Once we got me into bed, Pop helped me with water and pills and one last crack at the bedpan.

"Thanks for everything today, Pop," I said sleepily. "Goodnight. I love you."

"I love you too, Kim."

At least that's what I assume he said, because I'm pretty sure that before he finished, I fell into a deep sleep into a dreamy place a million miles away. *This is going to be wonderful*, I remember thinking.

And wonderful it was—until it wasn't. Like clockwork, once the pain meds faded, I woke to the torment of muscle and bone spasms. I gently rubbed the pain sites to try to distract my central nervous system. It provided a little relief. Then I reached for the pain medicine and Zofran for nausea and swallowed both. The faintest light from the street glowed through the side windows on each side of the front door. I always said a prayer for relief when the intensity became this bad. *Lord Jesus, please take away my pain and someday use it for Your glory!*

I rocked back and forth, rubbing every site that throbbed in pain. I told myself that any diversion was good. That night, the agony was overwhelming. I begged for relief, but it wasn't coming. I groaned and whimpered aloud, knowing that no one could hear me. I felt so alone on nights like this in the hospital, and there at home, it was somehow worse, with my husband and children away, and Pop asleep upstairs. My mind wanted to sleep, but my body wouldn't permit it. Tears rolled over my cheeks, into my lap.

To distract myself, I remembered something my mom had told me about pain when I was a young girl. She said that labor, although very intense, was pain worth bearing. I never understood that until I was in labor myself, and then I got it. One look into the eyes of my infant children, and the pain fell away. I had to hold onto that now, to see this as a kind of labor. Because truthfully, some days I wanted to give up and die. When the pain was at its height, dying would have been the easiest thing in the world. But then I thought about my family—my husband and children and everyone else I loved—and I knew I couldn't give up; I couldn't stop trying to heal. I had to keep marching forward to look into the eyes of my children as they grew into the great people I knew they would become.

I didn't wake Pop that night. What else could he have done for me? This was my burden to bear, and with God's help, I would do just that.

I must have eventually fallen asleep, because in the morning I woke to more pain—pain, reprieve; pain, reprieve; pain, reprieve; lather, rinse, repeat. I didn't know how much longer I could do this. It was destroying me, little by little, gnawing at my sanity. *Please God, enough is enough!*

Every time I reached for the pills with a shaking hand, I remembered how hard I had fought for sobriety. I felt shame and guilt, as if I was betraying my sober self. I didn't ever want to be addicted again. The nurses and doctors told me not to worry, but I did worry. I'm an addict! Recovery was precious to me—it gave my life back to me—and every narcotics drip or pain pill felt like a relapse. I couldn't live without the pain meds. Wasn't that the definition of addiction? Intellectually, I knew the difference, but emotionally, I felt like I was failing. My mind played tricks on me. *Do I really need that pill, or do I want it? Take it! No, don't take it!* It felt like a battle between good and evil, between angels and demons. I was playing with the pills in my hand, shaking them like dice. Was I gambling with my sobriety? Suddenly, I was hit with a wave of spasms that took my breath away. Without thinking any more about it, threw the pills into my mouth and washed them down, swallowing hard against the gag reflex it always triggered. Instantly, I felt ashamed, like I had fallen off the wagon. Was there any other way to relieve the pain? I knew the answer to that one.

I heard the shower running upstairs, then the welcome sound of his feet on the stairs. Sometimes the pain was more bearable when

I wasn't alone. I blotted my eyes dry, but continued to writhe. I worried I had waited too long to take the pills—that I had missed the window, and the pain wouldn't go away. That was how my mind worked those days.

"How are you this morning?" Pop greeted me.

"Not good," I said, my voice raspy. "I'm having so much pain, and nothing's helping yet."

"What can I do? Should I call a doctor?"

"No, nothing. I just have to ride it out." I winced, and then said, "I don't know how much more I can take! This sucks."

"I know it does," Pop said gently. "I know it does. How about one of those scrambled eggs you love?"

"Not yet. But you go ahead. Have some coffee at least."

Pop returned with his coffee. I rubbed my legs, and the pain finally eased a bit. "It's finally getting a little better. Maybe I'll take that coffee now." *I'm going to conquer this damn pain yet!*

Pop returned and handed me a cup of coffee. The aroma tickled my nose with delight. The hot liquid on my tongue was sweet and creamy the way I liked it, but not too sweet or too creamy. *This is home,* I sighed. "Maybe I am ready for one of those scrambled eggs, but only one, please, and nothing else."

After I surprised myself by devouring the egg, Pop brought me a basin of warm water along with my toiletries and a clean set of pajamas. By the time I finished bathing, the pain was tolerable. I swam in the wonderful feeling of being clean and as close to pain free as I got those days. Tired from the morning's efforts, I fell asleep quickly and slept for several hours.

Rod and the kids called later as they got ready for the beach. I could hear by the excitement in their stories that they were having fun. Rod said we could expect them home by nine that night, and they were bringing goodies!

Shortly after that call ended, the phone rang again. Pop took the call, spoke in a friendly way for a bit, then handed me the portable phone. I assumed it was a friend or family member by the way he was talking. It was Dr. Yue, my orthopedic surgeon from Yale New Haven. He said he was visiting his mom nearby and would I mind if he visited? He wanted to see how I was doing at home.

I couldn't really say no. I gave him the address.

Pop and I were speechless. What doctors did house calls anymore? Dr. Yue was one of a kind!

Before too long, the doorbell rang. Madison ran to the door barking before Pop could get her, but he caught up to her and grabbed her by the collar, then opened the front door.

I could see the front door from my bed. Pop and Dr. Yue introduced themselves. Then I called out, "Hi Dr. Yue. What a nice surprise!"

He walked towards me, but Madison broke away from Pop and headed straight for the young doctor. For a moment, I thought Madison was going to tackle him, but Dr. Yue stopped in time and let Madison sniff at his million-dollar hands. He must have passed the test. When I called Madison to me, she returned to my bedside.

Dr. Yue snapped on some gloves and unwrapped my lower right leg, which was known as "Dr. Yue's leg" at the hospital, since he worked on that leg almost exclusively. "Your right leg and foot look really good. Your incision is healing without signs of infection. The drainage looks good. Now let's take a look at the left."

"But that's Dr. Shin's leg," I protested. That leg needed the expertise of a plastic surgeon—Dr. Shin. "He's very serious about that!"

"That's okay, I just want to take a quick look." When the dressing was off, he frowned in disbelief. I could see for myself that a dime-sized hole exposed my leg down to the tibia. "I have to get in touch with Dr. Shin immediately. You need to get back to the hospital. If that opening isn't closed quickly, you'll lose the leg!" He plucked his pager from his belt and paged Dr Shin. Then he rewrapped the right leg while Pop held it up.

His beeper chirped, and he called Dr. Shin. When he finished the call, he said, "Dr. Shin's going to make the arrangements to get you back to the hospital as soon as possible. Realistically, it probably won't be until tomorrow morning since it's Sunday. I'm so glad I listened to the voice in my head telling me to pay you a visit. I'm sorry your time at home was cut short, but this is serious. Very serious. There's nothing you'll need to do. The hospital will notify the agencies. The social workers will contact the ambulance service and let you know the pick-up time. Have you had a fever?"

"No, I haven't."

"Let us know immediately if that happens, okay?"

"I will."

"See you back at the hospital," he smiled grimly, shaking Pop's hand before he left.

"I'll let Rod know," Pop said to me after he saw Dr. Yue to the door. "I'll call from Rod's office."

"I'll talk to him later, when we know more," I said. *Well that was a short visit home*, I thought. For all my fears about coming home, now that I was there, I didn't want to leave.

I was depressed and didn't have much interest in eating the lunch Pop thoughtfully made for me. Rod and the kids were skipping the beach that day to come back early. I felt bad about that, but at least I'd get to spend time with them before I left.

....

CHAPTER 27

SURGERY AND FIREWORKS

Mid-morning Monday the ambulance arrived at the house to take me back to the hospital. I prayed I wouldn't let fear overtake me on the drive. It was still so new to be outside where I felt this vulnerable. As we headed down Georges Hill Road, my heart raced as fear set in. This ambulance had windows, too, open to all those dangerous drivers in their dangerous vehicles. And then it came to me, a simple solution. What if I just closed my eyes?

The forty-five-minute ride went quickly with my eyes closed. When we arrived, my old room was taken, so they put me in another private room closer to the nurses' station. It was Brooke's day off, so I was admitted and cared for by another nurse.

Rod, Pop, and the kids arrived just before Dr. Shin and his partner. They too, were upset with the hole in my leg, though I wondered why no one had caught it before. None of the skin grafts had taken, Dr. Shin explained. There wasn't enough blood circulation.

Then he explained the procedure. "We're going to bring muscle and artery graft transfers to your left lower leg. That's why we're including an artery—to provide blood to the muscle graft."

"How long will it take?" Rod asked.

"It's a very long surgery, so if I was you, I wouldn't wait at the hospital. I'd estimate at least twelve hours, maybe longer. She'll go to Intensive Care overnight and then return here the next day, barring any complications."

Rod looked as discouraged as I felt. *Twelve hours? What the hell was going to take them so long? I'll be puking for days after all that anesthesia.*

Then the doctor turned to me and said, "I'd like to look at your abdomen for a potential muscle flap harvest site." He lifted my gown to reveal my stomach. "No, that won't work. May we look at your back?"

"Sure," I said. I sat forward, and they untied the gown to expose my back. "We could harvest a flap from right here." He touched an area my bra crossed. When I told him that, he tied the closure at my neck and thought some more. "Suppose we harvest the left radial artery and the small muscle flap in her wrist," he said, then asked me, "Are you right-handed?"

"Yes."

"The left arm then. Do you have any objections to us using your left forearm?"

"No, I don't."

"Your surgery is scheduled for six tomorrow morning. The nurses will wake you up around four to get you ready, so get some extra rest today. It'll last at least until six in the evening, possibly even later. It's a very tedious, delicate surgery, all done under magnification. You probably won't be awake until you get to ICU. Do you have any questions?"

"No," I said quietly.

"I'll mark your arm tomorrow, just before you go in. We'll see you then, bright and early."

The rest of the day after they left I obsessed about the long surgery ahead of me. I couldn't help but think about the pain and nausea I faced on the other side. It was difficult to stay positive when one thing after another kept going wrong.

Pop's wife, Cee Cee, was flying into Philly the next day, and Pop was going to drive to the airport to pick her up. Rod and the kids planned to go to the shore for the Fourth of July holiday. Pop and Cee Cee were staying in Connecticut and planned to visit me daily. I was excited to see Cee Cee again. She was a lot of fun to be around—we giggled over the silliest of things. She was definitely good therapy!

Fourth of July is my second favorite holiday, just behind Christmas. Ever since I was a small child, fireworks thrilled me with their cascade of colors and the loud booms that drilled right through me. I had seen my first fireworks at the White House while we were stationed at Fort Lee in Virginia. You'd think I would have been disappointed by every display after that, but no, I loved every single one of them. I was still a little girl at heart when it came to fireworks. Even sparklers thrilled me! I grew sad that this would be the first year I couldn't see fireworks.

Four in the morning arrived all too soon when the overhead lights flashed on and the nurse called me by name. "It's time to get you ready for surgery," Brooke said.

"Okay," I said, happy that Brooke was back at least.

For the next hour and a half, my room was a flurry of activity. At exactly five-thirty, the transporter arrived to take me to the operating room. I kissed Rod goodbye. I tried not to be hypervigilant with all the activity in the hallways. Before long, a peace came over me as the familiar smell of the OR enveloped me. My friend Shep was the nurse anesthetist. "We'll give you everything in our arsenal to prevent post-op nausea and vomiting," he said. "I just started to push your anesthesia. We'll take good care of you, Kim. Goodnight." That was the last thing I heard.

It was around eight-thirty at night when my eyes opened to someone calling my name in the recovery room. I fell back to sleep while the nurses completed their initial assessment. When I fully woke up, the queasiness hit me. I asked for Zofran for the nausea. I also felt something strange in my foot. "Why is my left heel burning? It feels like someone started a fire beneath it."

The nurse looked at my heel, then said, "I don't see anything."

I moved in and out of awareness for the next hour or so. Then one of the nurses announced, "We're taking you to the ICU now."

"Okay," I croaked. My throat was sore and chapped from the tube snaking there during surgery. I was so drugged up I didn't even worry about the nurses pushing my bed through the hallways to the ICU. We went through the doors into an all too familiar setting for me. This time I was in the bed, instead of running around assessing my own patients. I preferred the latter!

Once the nurses assessed me, Rod was permitted to see me. They let him stay for the night in a chair that opened into a bed, complete with linens and pillows from a nearby cupboard. I had Rod look at my burning heel several times, but he didn't find anything either. Eventually, one of the aides velcroed sheepskin foot coverings on both feet.

That didn't help much. That night was a cascade of pain, retching, vomiting, more pain, and little sleep to provide relief. By morning rounds, I no longer felt like a human being. I felt like a wild, wounded, caged animal, tormented by her captivity.

Back in my room on the seventh floor, I prayed I didn't need too many more surgeries, especially those as long as yesterday's.

Dr. Shin and his residents visited and seemed happy with the results. He explained the burning in my heel as possible nerve damage from the surgery. Only time would tell. That was easy for him to say.

I dozed briefly until Pop and Cee Cee arrived. They had a surprise for me. "I know how much you like fireworks," Cee Cee said. "So I did a little research, and I found that we'll be able to see New Haven's fireworks from your windows. I'll bring a picnic! How does that sound?"

"That's so thoughtful. I thought for sure I'd miss them this year. You're a genius, Cee!"

For the rest of the day, we visited when I wasn't dozing off from the Dilaudid. The next day the kids and Rod were leaving for Wildwood. The Fourth was on Thursday, and they planned to return to Connecticut

Sunday evening. It would be nice for them to get away, since their last trip was cut short. The fireworks at the shore were always beautiful and worth the wait.

Rod went home that night once I went to sleep so he could get packed for the weekend. They stopped by on their way to New Jersey the next day to say good-bye. I was glad they were going. I didn't want to be the fun killer. And they were happy that Cee had thought of a way for me to see fireworks.

I spent the day in anticipation, and finally, just in time for my growing appetite, Cee and Pop bustled into the room. Cee unpacked the huge picnic basket, a real Fourth of July feast—pulled pork on Ciabatta rolls, potato chips, iced tea, and brownies for dessert. She also brought red, white, and blue paper plates and napkins!

The evening was punctuated by laughter amidst pain. Pop and Cee Cee helped me get comfortable as best they could, and helped me with the pain medicine when necessary. I dozed at times while we waited. The show was slated to begin at nine sharp. Cee made sure I was awake just before nine, but nothing happened. All we saw was an empty sky. I could tell that Cee Cee was worried that she had gotten it wrong and was about to disappoint me. Finally, about a half hour later, the first of the fireworks exploded in the night sky. My bed was too far away from the window to see fully. Between explosions, Cee Cee and Pop unlocked the bed and moved it closer to the window. I could see everything from there, one huge colorful explosion after another. As I did as a small child, I gasped with every explosion. One seemed better than the next, but it had been a long couple of days, and I fell asleep before it ended! Pop and Cee quietly said their goodbyes after returning the bed to its proper position.

Dr. Shin told me the next morning that sometime the following week I'd be transferred to the hospital's rehabilitation unit—the one for physical therapy, not addiction. His team was pleased with the surgical outcome. The pulses in my left leg were stronger now. I still hadn't seen the harvest site on my wrist, but they didn't plan to remove that dressing for another ten days. In rehab, I would learn how to be more independent—to use a wheelchair by myself, take care of myself in the bathroom, and so on.

When I told him the news on the phone, Rod was excited. It meant I was making progress, even though at times it didn't seem that way.

CHAPTER 28

PHYSICAL REHABILITATION

I t was tough saying goodbye to all of the special nurses and aides that had taken care of me during the three-month stay on the seventh floor. I will always remember Brooke, Christina, Joe, Debbie, and Megan, and how much they all helped me on this healing journey. Rod brought in food and goodies for all three shifts as a thank you. They were all grateful and teary-eyed and promised to come see me once I was transferred.

I realized that I had much to learn before I'd be able to do anything independently. I had been confined to bed for so long I lost most of my muscle tone. Those ten plus years as a runner meant nothing now! The simplest of things made me short of breath. I was debilitated, emaciated, and weak. I had worked hard to be in such good health, but over the past three months all of my strength and energy had gone into saving my life! Now, I'd have to work hard to get back in shape! It was tough to accept. I had fought so hard the last three months, but here I still faced an uphill battle.

I'd be in rehab for approximately two weeks. Then maybe I could go home permanently. That sounded good to me. I couldn't wait to sleep in my own bed (though I wouldn't be able to do that until I could get up and down the stairs). I felt like a child again; I had so much to relearn.

While in rehab, I took Physical Therapy and Occupational Therapy. I also had a roommate, so Rod went home each evening. I worked on endurance by sitting in the wheelchair instead of the bed. The door to the bathroom was wide enough to accommodate the wheelchair, and it was large enough inside for me to maneuver around as needed. I couldn't get my right leg wet, so my only option was to wash at the sink.

I wasn't allowed to put weight on my right leg either since I had an Ilizarov external frame attached to it. The Ilizarov looked a bit like a cylindrical cage attached to the leg by spikes. Its purpose was to keep the leg bones in place while I regrew the seven centimeters of bone I lost in the accident. This contraption could be dangerous at night since the spikes stuck out from the cage and were long enough to stab my left leg if I wasn't careful. I wrapped an egg crate and sheepskin around the spikes for protection.

I was able to get out of bed to my wheelchair without help, but I'd get short of breath and have to rest and catch my breath before I could do anything else. I could also wheel myself into and out of the bathroom without help, but I'd need to rest right afterwards. Even during my bath, I'd stop every so often to slow down my breathing. Everything I did was designed to increase my independence. I got back into bed after lunch for a nap. By then I was exhausted! I had to conserve energy when possible.

Dressing myself was difficult, but the occupational therapist provided me with adaptive equipment to make it easier. Each day, I learned more advanced exercises. My progress was steady. I always pushed myself to do more and learn more.

One day, I had PT in the PT room instead of my own hospital room. Megan, the physical therapist, had me try to stand between the parallel bars and support myself with my hands and arms. I wasn't sure I could, but I did it!

Then she said, "Take a few steps."

"What?" I said. "Are you sure?"

She nodded.

I was even less sure about this, but I summoned every bit of strength and willpower I had, and I did that, too! It was more stumbling than steps, but I was as proud of myself as if I had just run five miles.

Megan clapped, then announced, "I'm calling Dr. Yue!"

In a few minutes, Dr. Yue walked into the center. I was sitting in my wheelchair to rest.

"Can I do a few more?" I looked from Megan to Dr. Yue.

"I'd love to see that!" Dr. Yue smiled broadly.

I pushed off the arms of the wheelchair to stand up, my arms shaking with the effort. Megan stayed behind me with the wheelchair. I grabbed the parallel bars for balance, then slowly and ever so carefully, moved one foot in front of the other one, taking small but deliberate steps. I was doing it! After three months in bed, I was walking! My smile was huge and mirrored by Megan and Dr. Yue. I teared up I was so happy and excited.

"That's amazing!" Dr. Yue said. "Thanks for paging me, Megan. Keep up the good work Kim!" he said, then turned to leave.

"I will!" I sat down in the wheelchair. By the look of astonishment on his face, I wondered if he thought I was ever going to walk again. I wasn't sure how I felt about that.

I still had the dressing on the donor site on my left arm until one morning Dr. Shin and his residents arrived very early and told me it was finally time to remove that dressing. They peeled it away one layer at a time, exposing a deep purple scar.

"That looks great," Dr. Shin announced.

What? I yelled in my head, staring at the half-inch deep gouge in my wrist. *Is he out of his damned mind?* Plus, a painful neuroma bulged out at my wrist, and they weren't sure what they could do to free up the entangled nerves. More surgery to consider. I was sick with the news.

Before long, they had all scurried out of the room and off to their next assignment. I sat in bed and cried and cried and cried. I felt like a science experiment gone off the rails. It was bad enough to have such awful scars on my legs, but now I had one on my wrist, and the nerve damage was extremely painful. One step forward and two steps back. Ten steps back! How was I going to hide this scar? I'd never be able to wear a watch or bracelet on my left wrist again. It would be too painful. I cried, and wept, and sobbed, feeling very sorry for myself. Looking back, given what I had been through with my legs, this shouldn't have been that big a deal. I mean, if I had to have that scar to save my leg, that was worth it, right? But I was worn out and ragged, on my last nerve, exhausted, emotionally and mentally. To me, right then, it was a big deal.

I called Rod, but I sobbed so hard he had a tough time under-standing me. "I have a horrid scar on my wrist and the nerve pain is dreadful. I'm so sad and disappointed. I'll never be able to hide it!"

"It's okay. Kim. It's okay. I'm on my way. Kim, I love you no mat-ter how many scars you have. You're alive and you have your legs. I'll always be grateful for that!"

"That's easy for you to say. You don't have to look at my scars twen-ty-four seven!"

"I know, I know. I don't. And I don't want to minimize how you feel. But what I do know is that I love you and that you're beautiful inside and out. Don't give up hope, my love. It may not seem like it, but you're getting there."

I wheeled into the bathroom to do my bath, but when I accidently hit my left wrist on the sink, the nerve pain shot through me like I was being electrocuted. I couldn't do anything but hold my wrist and cry.

Nothing I did made it better. I sat in my wheelchair and held my wrist for the longest time, sobbing in disbelief. *I'm a freak of a science experiment, nothing more. I should've died. Why didn't I just die? This is more than anyone should ever have to deal with.*

Then by force of habit, I finished in the bathroom and made my way back to bed to face the rest of the day. What else was I going to do?

CHAPTER 29

GOING HOME FOR GOOD

True to their word, after two weeks in rehab and three-and-a-half months in the hospital altogether, they were sending me home. And I was ... happy? Ecstatic? Overjoyed? I knew I should have been all these things, and to some degree I was, but I was also flat-out terrified. It hadn't gone so well the last time we tried this, and that had been for only three days!

It was the little things and the big things. PTSD was clearly still an issue that would require years of therapy to overcome. I felt safer in the hospital, with doctors, nurses, and therapists available twenty-four seven. What would it be like at home? Would I be able to advocate for myself?

And sure, everything at home had been planned and put in place for my care. The hospital bed with the air mattress awaited my return, and appointments with visiting nurses, counselors, and physical therapists were set up. Rod and the social worker figured out all of the details. But the bed was still in the dining room and offered only limited privacy. I was still in pain a good deal of the time, and I cried, and groaned, and sometimes screamed. And that was on a good day.

I didn't want the kids to see that. How long before they'd resent me and beg for their real mother back?

It wasn't rational, I know. They were good kids (still are!), but there's nothing rational about PTSD. There's no explaining it away. My fears were as real to me as my hand in front of my face.

And there was another fear I couldn't tell anyone about—Rod was driving me home. Rod—my loving, supportive, superhero rock-star of a husband, who had proved his love and compassion over and over again since my accident—was an awful, aggressive driver, the kind who tailgated the car in front of him to go faster, the kind who veered from lane to lane to gain a car-length advantage, the kind who sped up to a red light and took off at a green light like he was in a drag race. Driving with him had terrorized me *before* the accident. And now I hyperventilated rolling down the hallways in my hospital bed. I couldn't tell Rod, though. He was so elated to be the one bringing me home. I didn't want to hurt his feelings. The way I felt had nothing to do with him or the kids. It was all because of my own super-heightened fears of reinjury!

I knew Megan, my physical therapist, would be assisting me into the back of our Suburban. And Rod had told me he was removing a middle seat and would bring a bunch of pillows to accommodate my extended legs. But none of these preparations allayed my fears at all.

The discharge was planned for just after lunch. My stomach hurt, and I could barely eat anything. The nurse came in just after lunch to go over the discharge plans. Rod had already moved me out—taken home my cards and the still salvageable flowers. Then she paged Megan to let her know that we were ready to go home. Megan wheeled me downstairs where Rod had been instructed to park. It was bittersweet to say goodbye to the nurses and therapists. Many of them had become friends. I was teary eyed as we approached the elevator.

Beforehand, Megan and I had rehearsed the procedure for getting into the vehicle. I gave it all that I had, and it went smoothly, just as Megan had described. Once inside, though, I had to catch my breath.

My poor little heart felt like it was pounding out of my chest. I was belted in and as ready as I'd ever be.

As I feared, Rod hadn't changed his driving style since I'd been gone. The tailgating shouldn't have surprised me, or the aggressive passing. Every driver in front of him was wrong in some way. As he zoomed by them, he'd sneer, "Let's see what an asshole looks like." Sometimes in the past this had been mildly amusing, but not that day.

"Rod, you're scaring me. Please stop driving like that. I'm serious!"

"I'm not doing anything wrong! That's how I drive. Close your eyes until we get home if it bothers you that much."

We all have our blind spots and this was Rod's. Nothing I could ever say would convince him that he was anything but the world's best driver. For most of the forty-five minutes of hell, as I called it in my head, I followed his advice and closed my eyes to go to my happy place. When the Suburban slowed to a gentle stop, I knew we had arrived safely! My panic drained away.

Rod brought my wheelchair to the passenger door and locked it into place. After removing the side piece from the wheelchair, I slipped my transfer board between the vehicle and the wheelchair, gradually lowering myself onto the floor next to the board. Then ever so slowly I scooted across the board and onto the wheelchair as Rod helped me with my legs. "That went perfectly, as if we had practiced it a million times!" I said to make up for my nervousness in the car.

Rod smiled as he closed the car door before unlocking the wheelchair and heading for the front door. The kids were in charge of Madison until I was safely inside. *I can't wait to see her again.* I got my wish sooner than I thought I would. The second Rod opened the front door Madison ran towards me as if she was going to jump in my lap. So much for the kids taking charge of her. Rod stopped Madison before she got to me, though, while I braced myself for disaster. Then he walked her towards me, lurching in excitement. She gave me kisses when she got to me. The kids were just as happy to have me home again, but were a little more restrained in their affection, giving me a kiss on the cheeks and a pat on the arm.

Once we were in the house, Rod pushed me over to the three large dining room windows, saying something about a surprise. And it was a surprise, a wonderful, beautiful surprise. The Southbury Garden Club had planted a flower garden of my favorite perennials just outside the windows in full view of my bed. They varied in height and color and surrounded a small pond in the yard—yellow, pink, and orange day-lilies, purple irises and asters, white peonies, bleeding hearts. I can't remember them all. As beautiful as they were, though, I couldn't give them the attention they deserved. I was suffering too much pain and anxiety.

I was so touched by their generosity, though, and their commit-ment of time and talent. That's what I really remember. One of the teachers I worked with planned to weed and prune the flowers all summer so they would continue to bloom.

The families in our town had done so much for me and my family. I had a list of all of those who had supplied a meal, bought gift cards to restaurants, and any number of other acts of kindness. I hoped to send a thank you card to all of them.

My pain wasn't too bad, but by the following morning, instead of looking out my windows and enjoying the brilliantly colored flowers on display, I looked up and saw the contrails the planes were leaving in the sky above our house and freaked out. *What if a plane crashes into our house? I'm stuck here. I couldn't get out by myself. Rod's got to call the police and fire and rescue crews and tell them I can't get out of the house by myself!* Part of me knew this was the PTSD talking, but the other part of me feared I was in grave danger and was scared to death. I couldn't focus on anything else. These thoughts bounced around my head. I lay in bed staring at the sky as my heart pounded. *I was afraid in the car, and now I'm afraid in my house!*

As soon as Rod came downstairs, I explained my fears and asked him to call the police station as well as the ambulance association and the fire company. He said he would, but I never followed up. I just assumed he took care of everything. I rested easier, knowing I'd be safe in my home. I felt better once I had a plan of action.

I felt I had little privacy in the hospital bed downstairs. Eventually, Rod would carry me upstairs at night, so I could sleep beside him. The first night we tried it, my PTSD got out of control until we reached the top of the stairs safely. After that, it got easier each night, and I did feel better sleeping in my own bed. We kept the bed downstairs for easy access during the day for the visiting nurses and the physical therapists.

Two psychotherapists also came to the house several times a week to counsel me and Adam. We learned that Adam felt responsible for my accident because he and Sarah had been fighting in the car. Therapy helped him learn that an accident is just that—an accident and no one's fault!

The therapists told me another interesting observation Adam had shared with them. They had asked him this question: "If you look at your life before your mom's accident and now, how would you compare the two?" Adam said he thought that life was much better now because we knew one another on a much deeper level. I had never considered that, but the more I thought about it, the more I agreed. They had all seen my vulnerability as well as my tenacity in wanting to be well again, no matter what that looked like. It was like the two sides of a coin; I certainly always wanted the heads-up side of the coin. Forward progress, always striving to get well. But knowing that my family was also seeing the tail side of the coin humbled me. If they could love that side of me, well, I had everything to be grateful for. Life was indeed good!

+ + +

That Christmas of 2002 we decided to go to Pennsylvania to stay with my parents through the holiday season. Because we weren't going to be home Christmas day, and, let's face it, because of the accident and my convalescence, I was planning to scale back my decorating that year. I usually did it up big—multiple Christmas trees covered in the ornaments I had begun collecting as soon as Rod and I got married; yards and yards of garland; dozens of figurines (Santa's and toy soldiers and manger scenes); wreathes and posters and stickers galore. The kids were having none of it, though. "You can't do that," they protested. "You can't change Christmas!" as if I was joining forces with the Grinch.

All right, I said to myself. *They've been through enough.* I dug in deep to give them the best Christmas I could. From my wheelchair, I put up every decoration and every artificial tree we had stored away. Standing briefly at times to reach the high spots. The house looked amazing. I baked cookies and made my famous chocolate covered pretzels, chocolate-covered peanut butter balls, and a variety of other candies as well. We had lots of treats for everyone on our Christmas list. I'm glad I made the effort, not only for the kids, but also for myself. It gave me something to do, helped me feel a bit like my old self.

Knowing how much I enjoyed Christmas, Rod took me to the Berkshire Mall to see what they had done that year. After pushing me through the entire mall, we made our way back to the center where they had set up a huge tree decorated in silver and gold.

"Do you want to people watch for a while?" he asked.

I didn't get out much, so I thought that might be nice. We sat for several minutes when one of the shoppers caught my eye. She was nimble and graceful as she balanced a load of packages and made her way from store to store, at one point stopping on a dime in front of a showroom that had caught her interest, then spinning away in the opposite direction, as if it had been choreographed—all without losing a single package.

"Rod, did you see that lady?" I tapped Rod's arm with the back of my hand then pointed.

"What lady?" he said, stretching to look where I was pointing.

"She's gone into the crowd," I said.

"What did I miss?"

"She was walking so gracefully, like she was dancing, and carrying all these packages. I'm never going to walk like that again, am I?" I said, dejected.

"Sure you will, someday. We'll have you dancing in no time," he said, trying to keep it light.

"Doubtful," I said. I couldn't imagine walking so freely again. It seemed impossible. Everyone in the crowded mall was walking better than I ever would, and that was taking me to a dark place. "I'm getting tired," I said. "Can we go now?"

✦ ✦ ✦

We stayed with my parents about five days on both sides of Christmas day. At that point, I was still using a wheelchair. Rod had to take me backwards down their steep driveway to get me inside the lower level, where we had a bedroom. During the day, he wheeled me up the steep driveway and to their front porch where I had to lift myself and scoot inside the first floor. Then Rod would bring my wheelchair inside and I'd have to use my arms to boost myself back into the wheelchair. It was hard work but the only way to get around. I'd go upstairs in the morning, and I'd stay there until I went to bed. It was too hard to do anything else.

I didn't do the Christmas shopping after my accident. Rod had to do it all. I was just too sick to participate. Decorating and baking was about all I could manage. Everyone tried hard to make this an exciting Christmas, but we were all a little subdued. My parents couldn't get over the shape I was in. They didn't know where to look when they talked to me, or what to talk about for that matter.

Many of our other relatives saw me for the first time that visit as well. Later, they told me they were speechless when they saw me. My injuries were very graphic.

The kids tried to have a good time—they were kids after all, and they still got presents, but their hearts weren't fully in it. We all had a patch of the post-holiday blues when we returned.

CHAPTER 30

CHALLENGES AND MORE CHALLENGES

We had enrolled both kids in the public school in the fall of 2002, even though Adam had been accepted at the Taft School, a private prep school in Watertown, Connecticut. For the sake of family sanity, we decided not to send him there. It would have been a logistical nightmare getting both kids to different schools, and we had enough pressures.

Rod had also tried to return to work after his leave of absence, but he found he had difficulty concentrating on anything but me. And because I needed him at home, he couldn't really travel as much as the job demanded. Eventually, he decided it was in the best interests of our family and the company that he give up his position. He worked out a severance package, and his career in Connecticut ended.

Unfortunately, he had to keep working to pay for my medical care. My medical bills were paid by my insurance, which I contributed to through Gainfield School. That coverage ended about one year after the accident, at which point I acquired insurance under the Consolidated Omnibus Budget Reconciliation Act, also known as COBRA. COBRA gave me the right to continue the same insurance as long as I paid the full premiums. When COBRA ended, I officially went on disability and paid the premiums through Medicare.

Because Rod's job no longer tied us to Connecticut, and with everything else going on, by the end of the 2002–2003 school year, we had decided to sell our house and return to Pennsylvania where we'd have a much larger support system. Besides, the cost of living in the southeastern portion of the state was a heck of a lot more reasonable than Connecticut.

Rod brought the two kids downstairs where I was sitting in my wheelchair. This was after Christmas.

"We've got something big to tell you," Rod began to an apprehensive look from the kids. He jumped right into it. "For the good of the family, Mom and I decided we're going to sell the house and move back to Pennsylvania."

"What?" Sarah shrieked. "I don't want to move!"

"Me either!" said Adam.

This wasn't going the way we had planned. "It was a decision we had to make," I explained. "Especially since Dad no longer has a job here."

"Well, I'm not moving!" Sarah spouted.

"Sarah, you have no choice, really. We're your parents, and it's our call. We thought about it a lot, and this is best for all of us."

"I hate you guys!" Sarah hollered, then ran back upstairs to her room.

Adam just turned and walked away, letting his silence speak for him.

"That went well," I said to Rod.

"They'll come around," Rod said. "They have to."

The next few days were quiet around the house. We didn't say too much more to the kids, but we continued to make plans to return to Pennsylvania. The house had been newly built when we moved in, and we had made many improvements, including outside landscaping and two decks. The realtor we hired told us we should make enough on the sale to recoup our investments. Someone very close to us didn't want to sell the house, though. Long after the sale was closed, and we had already moved, I found out that Sarah and our neighbor's daughter, Lisa, had written a warning in Sarah's closet: DO NOT BUY THIS HOUSE! IT'S HAUNTED! When Sarah finally told me about it, I laughed hard. Oh, the innocent minds of children!

If we were going to uproot our lives, we were going to build the house of our dreams in Pennsylvania. The town was Sinking Spring, about seventy miles northwest of Philadelphia. We enlisted the children in the planning to help them come to terms with the move. We wanted a property with a walkout basement exiting to the rear. The entire house would be kid friendly, so the kids could entertain friends. Adam wanted a music room in the basement, in addition to a rec room, an exercise room, and a full bathroom. Slowly but surely we were winning the kids over.

Once school ended in the spring of 2003, we packed up the house and put everything except our clothing into storage. The new house would be completed in mid-November. We stayed in our home at the Jersey Shore for the summer, and when school started, we moved into the apartment in my parents' home.

After the kids started school, they thanked us for making the move. They both loved their new schools, and in no time, they both made many new friends. This helped the transition for me. When my kids were happy, I was happy. It was a four-hour trip back to my doctors at Yale-New Haven, but I only had to return every couple of weeks, and it was mostly highway driving. Sometimes Rod drove me and other times I'd drive alone and stay at either Carole's or Sue's for a night. Sue was another close friend.

By mid-November, we moved into our new house. From my wheelchair, I sewed the curtains, a project that gave me a sense of purpose. The house looked more complete every day.

Rod decided to simplify life and return to teaching until our kids graduated from high school. He started by substituting throughout the county, and by the fall of 2004, he was able to find a full-time teaching job in an alternative-education high school. He no longer had to travel all over the world. It was wonderful to have him home in the evenings.

After the Ilizarov frame was surgically removed in the Fall of 2003, I was finally permitted to bear weight on the right side only. I had regrown the seven centimeters of bone pulverized in the accident. It had been a painful process of re-breaking my tibia each day at multiple sites to pull down the soft bone and gradually lengthen my limb. Unfortunately, the doctor had removed the frame too soon, and my right leg had begun to bow. The bowing got so severe over time it required a different surgical procedure. The greater the bowing, the more intense the pain. One step forward and two steps back.

Dr. Yue turned my case over to Dr. Michael Baumgardner, who knew more about limb lengthening procedures, though he wasn't an expert, we found out the hard way.

I returned to Yale for the surgery to attach the Taylor Spatial Frame to my left leg, so I could begin the process of re-growing the tibia and spent several days in the hospital after the surgery. Sue volunteered to drive me back to Sinking Spring after I was discharged. She was fun and as spontaneous as I was. I wasn't surprised when we got off the highway to go to a huge bakery in Rye, New York. We loaded up on bread and pastries for the folks at home.

Once we arrived at our house, I decided to go upstairs to take a nap. From the kitchen, I stood up, but before I could sit onto the steps, I cried out in pain and fell back into the wheelchair. Later, I learned that when I put weight on the leg, the internal device holding my bones in place had failed, re-breaking my tibia at various places along the six pins. The device had been attached incorrectly.

The pain was intense, and my leg swelled into a football. Rod called the orthopedic resident at Yale, but he was told no one was available until Monday morning. By Saturday, we knew I couldn't wait two more days in this kind of pain. Rod called the resident again to tell him I was returning to the emergency room, and I'd be there in four hours.

The ride back to the hospital was tough. Sue drove again, and every bump in the road produced an intense, stabbing pain in my leg. It wasn't Sue's driving—it was the multiple fractures. As soon as I returned to the hospital, x-rays confirmed that the internal mechanisms of the external fixator had failed, fracturing my tibia at multiple sites. I would have to return to the OR for more surgery on Monday. In the meantime, I was given Dilaudid intravenously to control the pain, but it only took the edge off. I actually looked forward to going under anesthesia, so I'd be pain free, at least for a while.

Bright and early Monday morning, I returned to surgery. Dr. Baumgarten reattached the external fixator, correctly this time. In what was becoming a nightmare of repetition, I woke in the recovery room with intravenous Dilaudid for pain. I was told that the external fixator was now intact without issues. Easy for them to say.

I remained hospitalized for four days. Rod came to Connecticut to pick me up and take me back to Sinking Spring. Before I left, they gave me the computerized schedule to follow for limb-lengthening. I was to turn the struts in the morning, re-breaking my tibia at multiple sites, per the computer-generated schedule. Every two weeks I was supposed to return to be evaluated and obtain an updated computer program sheet.

We joked with one another, saying someday there would be light at the end of the long tunnel. The kids asked me to stop saying that, since it didn't seem true. They couldn't see a light at the end of the tunnel of my pain and suffering. It was very difficult for my family, especially the kids, to see me in excruciating pain all the time.

One day when I returned to Connecticut, I saw Dr. Yue instead of Dr. Baumgartner. He said, "Kim, we are not limb-lengthening experts, and we've done our best, but we don't typically deal with Taylor Spatial Frames. You need to contact Dr. Dror Paley. He's the expert. He'll know better what to do. Make an appointment with him as soon as possible."

I thanked Dr. Yue for saving my life and limbs and told him that I'd never forget him.

When we got home, Rod located Dr. Paley at Sinai Hospital in Baltimore. The following day I called and made an appointment for Friday morning. My dad rode along with me, so Rod wouldn't have to take more time off school. (By then, Mom attended a senior day care for dementia, so she would be fine for the day.)

I didn't have any issues finding Sinai Hospital. It took me under two hours to get there, much easier than the drive to Connecticut. In the second-floor clinic, they took multiple x-rays of both legs and feet. Then we waited for five hours to see Dr. Paley.

Dr. Paley was mortified by the bowing in my right leg, and the way the external Taylor Spatial Frame had been attached, still incorrectly, according to him. "We are going to have to take that external fixator off your leg today. I'm hoping that some of the sites will heal before surgery next Tuesday. We will correct the bowing in your right leg as well as place another external limb-lengthening device on your left leg."

"Do you have an operating room available?"

"No, I don't have an operating room but my PA, Steve, can take the Taylor off here in the clinic." He indicated Steve, who was standing next to him.

"But it's bolted to my bones. Won't that be painful?"

"We can get pain pills for you to take before it's removed. We do that on kids all the time. You'll be good with two pills," Steve said.

"O-ka-ay," I said, ever the good patient. But I had my doubts.

My dad pushed me back to the waiting room, where we waited another two hours before the pain pills arrived. About thirty minutes later, Steve found me and wheeled me into the treatment room. I was so nervous and once on the table, I realized that Steve didn't even have power tools for the removal of the fixator attached to my bones. He described how he was going to attach the T tool to the strut and then hit the tool to break the strut away from the bone at all six locations.

"Okay, but if I ask you to stop, please stop immediately."

"Okay, I'll do that. Are you ready?"

"Yes." Then with eyes bugging out of their sockets, I watched as he secured a T-shaped device over the first strut. Next with extreme force, he struck the right side of the T with his palm, breaking loose the strut. "Stop," I hollered and waited for the extreme pain to lessen. "Okay, you can keep going."

He backed the first long strut out of my leg. It was painful, but not as bad as when he broke the strut away from the tibia. The two pain pills did nothing, and there was no way in the world they could do this to children. They had shamed me into agreeing to this barbaric procedure. It took me all I had not to lose it on them. Those darn pain pills were as good as two farts in the wind.

Five more times, he broke the strut away from the bone. Each time I grabbed his hand and forced him to stop until the unthinkable pain eased. Then ever so cautiously, he unscrewed and backed the strut out of my bone and leg.

After he removed the external fixator, he applied sterile dressings over the old strut sites and wrapped my lower leg in an ace bandage. Then I was put into a full leg, half cast and my entire leg was wrapped in ace bandages. I wouldn't be able to drive back to Sinking Spring with one leg in a cast, and my dad couldn't drive because he was legally blind. I'd have to figure something out once I got back to the waiting room.

My brother, Kevin, and his family lived in Silver Spring, Maryland, about thirty-five miles from Baltimore. He agreed to pick us up when he finished work in Washington, D.C., but he wouldn't get to us until at least seven-thirty that evening. Rod and Adam could pick us up the next day. Meanwhile, Rod had to pick up my mom and bring her to our place after she got home from daycare, because she couldn't be alone overnight. We had opened the limb-lengthening clinic in the morning and didn't leave that evening until long after the clinic had closed. My father and I were exhausted and hungry by the time we got to Kevin's house.

Mid-morning on Saturday Rod and Adam arrived at Kevin's, and after getting my car from the parking lot at Sinai Hospital, we drove home. Sarah and my mom had stayed behind.

Bright and early Tuesday morning, Rod and I headed back to Sinai Hospital for my next surgery. They planned to cut my right tibia apart and apply another Taylor Spatial Frame in order to correct the bowing that had occurred when the external fixator was removed prematurely. My left leg would also require another Taylor Spatial Frame so I could successfully regrow my shortened tibia. Surgery was successful, and I woke up in the recovery room in pain despite the medication drip. I was so tired of pain. I prayed that someday it would be gone.

I wouldn't begin the limb-lengthening process for a few days, but at that time I'd be given a computerized two-week schedule of adjustments to the fixators, and every two weeks I'd return to the clinic for x-rays and a visit with Dr. Paley. It had been a long time since I had external fixators on both legs. It was extremely awkward, and hard to get used to again.

I was told it was okay to put weight on both legs and that I needed to begin physical therapy to work on muscle strengthening and balance issues. I went home several days after surgery and started PT immediately. Learning to walk with external fixators on both legs was a challenge because I had to keep my legs apart while throwing one heavily weighted leg forward at a time. I didn't have any stamina and became short of breath whenever I tried to walk. I spent most of the time in the wheelchair. My legs hurt too much to stand for any length of time.

✦ ✦ ✦

The physical toll from all the surgeries was great, but so was the emotional toll. With the fixators on my legs, I looked like some kind of cyborg from a sci-fi movie. When I was out in public, I naturally drew attention. Some people were simply curious, but others were downright rude. I could usually shrug off the attention, but I'm only human and sometimes it got to me.

One time, while still using a wheelchair, I went with Rod and Adam to the Lancaster Outlet Stores in Lancaster, Pennsylvania. It was a beautiful Saturday afternoon, and I gloried in the warmth of the sun on my face. We had visited nearly every store in the complex, but Adam and Rod wanted to check out one last store—the Bose Outlet. Electronics aren't my thing, so I told them, "I'll wait outside. Just wheel me off to the side. I'll be fine." They did what I asked and entered the store.

As I basked in the sun, two elderly couples strolled my way. *How nice*, I thought. *Good for them.* When they got within ten feet, the man in the lead looked me over and said, "What happened to you?"

His tone was borderline discourteous, but I was used to that. My response was brief. "I was in a car accident." I looked him in the eye and smiled.

"I hope the car doesn't look as bad as you do," he quipped. The whole group laughed loudly as they passed by.

How cruel! I thought, then sobbed. I couldn't help it. That's what all I had been through added up to for other people—a cause for laughter? After a few minutes, I quieted down and wiped away the tears. I didn't want to tell the guys what had happened.

I guess I couldn't hide it. The first thing Rod said when we met up was, "Why were you crying?"

"I wasn't crying," I lied.

"Kim, c'mon. It's me. I know you were crying. What made you cry?"

"Some old man. I told him I was in an accident, and he said he hoped the car doesn't look as bad as I do. Then his friends all laughed."

"What the hell? Where are they? Where'd they go?"

"That's okay. They're long gone. I took it hard, that's all."

"I'm so sorry, Kim. What a bunch of asses."

All the way back to Sinking Spring, I fell into a muck of self-pity, the man's comment tumbling in my head. *How can people be so cruel? I can't wait to get these fixators off, so no one will ever laugh at me again.*

Sometimes it went the other way, though, and my faith in humanity was redeemed.

The following weekend, Sarah and I were in Cape May shopping in the quaint Victorian shopping area with its cobblestone walkways. She wanted to go into a rather small clothing store, but I declined. "Sarah, the store is small and crowded and there's a huge bump at the door. It will be difficult to get my wheelchair in there."

"No, I'm taking you in. It'll be fine."

"Then put me in a corner where I'll be out of the way."

Once inside, she pushed me to the front corner, opposite the door, and left me there while she walked through the store, checking out the clothing on the shelves and hangers. After a few minutes, a young father and his young daughter, who I guessed was about four, came through the door. The second the little girl's eyes met mine, she tried to free her hand from her daddy's. The father wouldn't let go and repeatedly said, *No!* to the small, dark-haired girl. That didn't stop her from trying to get free. Finally the father released her. She came right to me.

"What happened to you?" she said in a soft, innocent voice.

I didn't want to frighten her, so I matched her soft tone and said, "I was in an accident, but someday I'll be fine."

Her eyes opened wide, and she took a step closer to me. "I'll pray for you."

"You're so sweet," I said. "Thank you. That's all I need." My eyes welled with tears, but this time they were tears of gratitude.

She went back to her father and took his hand again. The father turned to me and said, "I'm so sorry. She should know better."

"Oh, no. Don't be sorry. Your precious little girl just made my day!"

To this day I think of that little girl as another tiny angel among us.

CHAPTER 31

I'VE NEVER SEEN *THIS* BEFORE

As soon as school ended, we all eagerly piled into the car to head to the Jersey Shore for a summer of fun and sand-filled shoes. We loved to spend our days on the beautiful, white, sandy beach of Wildwood Crest.

When we got within forty-five minutes of the beach, the smell of brackish bay water always woke the sleepy dogs, Madison, the Weimaraner, and two dachshunds, Riley and Sadie. We'd laugh, and then I'd ask them in my talking-to-the-dogs voice, "Do you know where we're going now? Oh yes you do. Oh yes you do." They'd wag their tales and look at me with those doggy eyes as if to say, "Of course we do!" For the rest of the drive, they were on high alert. They even knew when we turned down the street we lived on, and were always the first ones out of the car, whether because they had to pee really bad or were excited to be there, I was never exactly sure.

As with every summer, guests came out of the woodwork, and we had many visitors. As soon as we arrived, we received daily texts with dates and names to add to the beach calendar. Everyone always hoped to get their first choice, but the calendar filled quickly. My friends knew that availability was limited and when a slot was full, I didn't allow others to visit at the same time. We also didn't want to fill each week with guests because it was our vacation time as well, and even though we liked to entertain, it wasn't fun every week. It was just too much work for me given my condition. Plus, I was certain I'd require more surgery in Baltimore.

When Carole and her kids visited, we always had fun, but one morning, when I was about to turn my fixator struts, I noticed that one of the large external rings that held the struts in place in the left fixator was cracked and ready to break. "Oh, dear God, Carole. Come and look at this."

Carole hurried to me. "You better get in touch with Dr. Paley right away. That ring looks like it's ready to snap!" she said.

"I've never seen anything like this." I grabbed my phone and called the clinic in Baltimore. When I told them what I noticed, they were shocked. They asked me to take a picture and email it to them. Within a minute, they called me back.

"Don't put any weight on your foot, get in the car now and come directly to the clinic." Then he added, "Dr. Paley has never seen anything like this."

Did they think that was reassuring?

"Never a dull moment with you," Carole said.

"I can use a few dull moments."

Carole drove my car while I rode in the passenger seat. It was a three-hour trip to Baltimore since we had to head northeast before we could turn southwest.

If I had to make this drive with anyone, Carole was a great choice. She has a dry sense of humor, and when we're together we laugh and laugh. She loves life, and she loves to eat. Whenever we hit the boardwalk, we start at Sam's Pizza then pick up Boardwalk Fries with malt vinegar and plenty of salt topped off with Kohr's frozen custard. You'd never know she was diabetic from the way she ate, but she always knew just how much insulin to inject. A little thing like diabetes wasn't going to stop her! She never had a dull moment of her own, either. We joke that she invented drive-through gas stations in Connecticut the time she drove away from the pump with the nozzle still in the tank, damaging her new car that she was filling up for a trip to see us in New Jersey.

This trip to Baltimore was uneventful, except we stopped three times for Carole's bathroom breaks. I was accustomed to waiting for hours before seeing Dr. Paley, but the second I arrived at the clinic, I was taken to a treatment room. Dr. Paley and two of his fellows came in to see me immediately. By now the titanium ring was almost severed.

"I've never seen anything like this," Dr. Paley announced, truly perplexed.

"So I gather," I said. "I have no idea when it happened. Everything was going fine, then this morning when I went to adjust the struts, I saw the crack. I couldn't believe it!"

Dr. Paley and the fellows talked softly to one another. I stopped listening when it was clear that not only couldn't I fully hear them, I also couldn't understand their jargon. Carole and I sat silently.

Dr. Paley turned to address me. "Okay, these two doctors are going to bolt another titanium ring above and below the broken ring. It's going to take a while because they have to be very careful. If anything moves, it will re-break the bone." Then he said, in a tone that seemed to be blaming me for something, "We've never done this before."

The fellows left and then returned with their arsenal of instruments and supplies. Over the next two to three hours, they worked at a steady pace, moving with precision, and discussing each move in advance. I was terrified that they had never done this before. Who wants to be a Guinea pig? I kept imagining the worst—that in the next second something would snap, and I'd experience tremendous pain. My heart raced, and I perspired profusely, especially when they seemed unsure of their next move.

In the end, they got it right, thank the Lord. They stabilized the broken ring with two additional titanium rings, and even if the first ring broke completely, the new rings would hold the fixator in place. I took a huge cleansing breath when they explained this to me. They followed up with x-rays, and after Dr. Paley evaluated the repairs, they said I was good to go.

After a quick bite to eat, Carole and I headed back to New Jersey, exhausted but relieved. I had dodged a bullet that day, perhaps more than one.

I had many more surgeries with Dr. Paley and his team over the next four years, twenty in all. At times the limb lengthening process was so painful I took narcotics like Morphine and Kadin. I was always very cautious with the narcotics, especially around the children, and I locked them in a safe in my bedroom closet. I didn't really think I had to worry about anyone getting into them, but as a mom and a nurse *Better safe than sorry* was my mantra. I hid the key in a different place every time, but sometimes I outfoxed myself and forgot where I hid it. This caused many a frantic search when the pain whelmed out of control, and I needed something that second.

CHAPTER 32

LOSE THE LIMP

My daughter Sarah has always been my toughest critic, but especially after the accident. She was twelve when the accident occurred, and when she was seventeen, I was still learning to walk again. One day she came home from school and said, "Mom, you need to lose the limp!"

"Are you serious, Sarah?" I looked down at my toes. "These legs are holding me up!"

"No, Mom. Lose the limp. It's embarrassing."

I was absolutely shocked, and my eyes filled with tears. *She's embarrassed? Really? What about me? I'm lucky I have the legs to limp on right now.* Did Rod and Adam feel the same way?

When Rod got home from work, I talked to him privately. "Do my scars or limp bother you?"

"No, why do you ask? I don't even see your scars, Kim. You have your legs! I'm in love with you because of who you are. Don't worry about your limp either. You're re-learning how to walk. Why do you ask?"

"Sarah told me to 'lose the limp' because it embarrasses her."

"Are you kidding me? I'll talk to her. Don't worry about it!"

"Don't be too rough on her. She might have a point."

The next morning, I had physical therapy. For me to use the car was an involved process. I wheeled myself to the rear of the car, stood up, hoisted the wheelchair into the cargo area, limped (as Sarah would say) to the driver's door, and swung myself into the seat. Once I was parked, I reversed the ordeal to get my wheelchair out of the car and head into the office. As soon as I saw Chris, my therapist, I asked him, "How can I lose my limp?"

"What are you talking about?" Chris said. "You're making good progress."

"I know, but Sarah said my limp is embarrassing!"

"Wow! She's a teenager, right?"

"Yeah, but still."

"Okay. Give me a minute to think about it! Go ahead and start your exercises."

Chris returned about forty-five minutes later. "Okay, I figured it out. You know your two front hip bones?"

"Yep."

"Pretend that your hip bones are headlights. Every time you take a step, lead with your hip and say to yourself, 'Headlight forward.' Say that with each step. Try it now."

I took several steps, holding my fists like head lights on my anterior hip bones as I repeated, "Headlight forward. Headlight forward."

"Say that every time you take a step."

And that was what I did. From that day forward, with every step I took, I said *Headlight forward* to myself. It became a habit, though no one else knew what I was doing. A full year later, I realized I wasn't saying *Headlight forward* any longer. I had officially lost the limp. Sarah was the first one I showed. "Sarah, watch this." I walked for her, about ten feet one way, then ten feet back.

"You don't limp anymore! I'm so proud of you, Mama!"

No model on a Paris runway could have been happier. That day I was grateful Sarah was my toughest critic! She pushed me to do something I might not have done on my own.

CHAPTER 33

THE END IS IN SIGHT ... OR IS IT?

Sarah graduated from high school in 2007 and chose to attend Arizona State University in Tempe, Arizona, to major in elementary and special education.

We had purchased a forty-five-foot-long Monaco Executive RV the year before. It had many bells and whistles and took us a while to get used to. Our training session before we took delivery was eight hours long! On our way home, we pulled up to a traffic light with our Jeep in tow, and we were longer than the eighteen-wheeler to our left! I said, "What the hell were we thinking?" We kept the RV in storage for a year, occasionally driving the forty-five minutes to the facility to start the engine, pull it out of the garage, then return it to the garage. We were too afraid to drive it any further.

In the summer of 2007, we screwed up our courage and planned a family RV trip to take Sarah to Arizona. The drive was long but uneventful, though we certainly got to know each other better in the small quarters. A few days after we arrived in Tempe, Adam returned to the east coast to go back to school at Lebanon Valley College where he was a music therapy major, and we stayed in Tempe for four to six more weeks, since Rod had retired a few months earlier.

It was incredibly hot in Tempe that summer and fall—we had six weeks of triple digit temperatures with little rain. But you know what? My legs felt so much better in that dry, desert climate. We sold the house of our dreams in Pennsylvania and bought a new one in Mesa, Arizona—far enough from ASU to give Sarah her independence, but close enough for her to come home for dinner and do her laundry every once in a while. We kept our beach house in Wildwood, though. We'll never give that up!

✦ ✦ ✦

Just over seven years after the accident I was scheduled for my last surgery with Dr. Paley. Dr. Paley had left his practice in Baltimore and opened another one in West Palm Beach, Florida, at St. Mary's Hospital. He planned to remove the last external fixator from my left leg as well as all the hardware that had broken off inside the leg over the years. I looked forward to not having fixators on my legs. It was a small thing, but my legs hadn't touched each other in years. The fixators had kept them apart. It was the normal things that most people took for granted that I longed for.

We had already moved to Arizona, but we were in Wildwood for the summer. I was going to catch a flight from Philadelphia to Orlando, where my step-mother-in-law, Cee Cee, was to pick me up and drive me the two-and-a-half-hours to West Palm Beach for the surgery. She lived in Kissimmee, about a half hour south of Orlando, and would stay in a hospitality suite until I was discharged.

The day before the flight, I was tired from the beach, so I changed into my pajamas earlier than most nights. I bent over to remove my sports bra and felt a lump under my right boob. I stood up to feel for it again, but it disappeared. I bent over again and found the lump, which had what felt like a tail. When I changed positions, it disappeared. *I had a negative mammogram three months ago*, I reminded myself. *It should be fine.*

I had Rod feel the lump just to be sure. "Yeah, there's a lump when you bend like that," Rod said. "You should call your gynecologist in the morning."

I went back upstairs to look over what I had packed for the trip. I tried not to worry, but my thoughts kept returning to the lump. *Damn, what if I have cancer! No, I can't. I can't think about it now. I'll call in the morning. It'll be fine.*

At nine the next morning, I called my doctor and explained what I found. He reminded me that the mammogram was negative. I told him about my surgery in Florida. He said we should repeat the mammogram and do an ultrasound the day I returned. That sounded like a reasonable plan to me. *One issue at a time*, I thought.

The surgery went as planned. It was great to wake up without anything but a dressing on my leg. I felt lighter—literally. Besides removing the fixator, Dr. Paley's team took out every broken screw left in my leg in the previous seven years. My post-operative pain level wasn't too bad. I only had to stay in the hospital for two days. Then Cee Cee and I returned to Kissimmee, where I recuperated four more days before returning to Philadelphia.

Rod picked me up at the airport, and we went directly to the appointment at the Reading Medical Center. I had a mammogram and an ultrasound of my breasts. Both were normal.

This was good news, great news even. I should have been celebrating. But I wasn't. Call it intuition; I knew something was still wrong. And I knew I should have the lump removed.

I talked to Rod, and he agreed. "Listen to your gut," he said.

I smiled grimly. "What's another surgery after fifty-one of them?"

The next morning, I called my gynecologist and asked him for the two surgeons he'd send his wife or daughter to for a lumpectomy. I chose Dr. Anna Shin (not related to Dr. Joseph Shin, the plastic surgeon who had worked on my legs) because she could get me in for the procedure in a few days.

Dr. Shin operated on August 24, 2009, in Reading. The surgery was no big deal compared to the leg surgeries. I went home the same day after waking up from anesthesia, and the pain was minimal. Dr. Shin removed the dressing the next day. It was almost over. We just had to wait for the biopsy results.

Four days later, Rod and I were driving to Philadelphia when my phone rang. It was Dr. Shin.

"Hi, Kim. I have your pathology report. Are you sitting down?"

It's never a good sign when your doctor asks if you're sitting down. "Yes. Go ahead."

"You have invasive ductal carcinoma, stage two. And apparently I didn't take a big enough margin around the lump. You need more surgery."

"Are you serious?" I said in disbelief. "Thank God I had you take it out! Can you please spell that for me? I'm a little dazed right now."

Slowly she spelled each word and I wrote the diagnosis on some scrap paper in my purse, my hand shaking. I looked at Rod and shook my head.

"Are you doing the surgery?" I asked Dr. Shin.

"No, you'll need a specialist. I'm referring you to Dr. Michael Brown. He's also at Reading."

She gave me the number. I wrote it on the same piece of paper, my eyes filling with tears, my mind a million miles away. She said good luck, and I thanked her. Then to Rod I said, "I can't believe it. Breast cancer! And just when I was about done with my legs. Thank God for my intuition. I could have been dead before I knew I even had it."

For the rest of the day, I was quiet and introspective. CANCER.

That night my emotions were raw, swinging in all directions. I wanted this cancer to be eradicated, no question. But did I have to lose my breasts? And hair, what about my hair? I was afraid of being further disfigured; my leg scars were horrific enough. As I drifted off to sleep, I prayed to God to help me cope and grant me peace.

The following morning, I made an appointment with Dr. Brown for the next week. Rod went along with me. We scheduled another lumpectomy for two weeks later, and I obtained a consult to the oncologist group. Dr. Brown performed the surgery as planned. He also removed the sentinel lymph nodes (the ones most likely to be infected by cancer) for analysis.

Now, it was a waiting game. By a week after surgery, the drainage was minimal, so Dr. Brown removed the drain. By the tenth day after surgery, the sutures were removed, as the incision had healed nicely. Next came the pathology report, which showed that the margin was clear of cancer cells; however, cancer cells were found in the lymph nodes. I had to discuss the findings with the oncologist.

I met with the oncologist, Dr. Leisure at Reading. I already knew I shouldn't do chemotherapy. When I was going through my leg operations, I had been infected with methicillin-resistant Staphylococcus aureus (MRSA) as well as Vancomycin-resistant Enterococci (VRE) and had part of my left tibia removed to fight them. These two organisms are likely to stay in my body forever. Since chemotherapy decreases the number of white blood cells (the infection fighters) in the body, if the MRSA or VRE infections returned after chemo, I wouldn't be able to fight them off and would likely die.

Dr. Leisure agreed with me, and we sought a second opinion at Johns Hopkins. Dr. Antonio Wolff at the Johns Hopkins Cancer Center was also concerned about the dangers of chemotherapy in my case. Before he made a decision, he requested an Oncotype DX test on the cancerous mass to determine how aggressive the cancer was. I bought a wig just in case. After several weeks, he told us my Oncotype number was a lucky thirteen. A score of 15 or less meant that the cancer was not very aggressive and wouldn't require chemotherapy. I couldn't have been happier. I'd probably have to have radiation, though, once I healed from surgery.

I was doing well enough for Rod and me to return to Arizona, where I would follow up with an oncologist and radiologist there. We planned to drive across country, taking a leisurely two weeks to make the twenty-five-hundred-mile trip.

When we were in Tennessee, I noticed fluid seeping from the surgical site, which had turned an angry red. When we stopped for the night, I tried to clean the site, but when I applied a gentle pressure, the wound ruptured and ejected a stream of thick pus, which projected across the room. I was mortified. Obviously, the wound was infected. The next morning I called Dr. Brown. He guessed I had a seroma, a buildup of fluid, that might be infected. He ordered antibiotics and told me to wrap my chest with an ace bandage as tightly as I could and see a doctor once I arrived in Arizona. With so many miles ahead of us and without any doctors to manage me once we arrived, it was unnerving to know that I had an infection in my chest so close to my heart and lungs.

By the time we arrived in Arizona, the infection had gotten much worse, and I felt sick. My oncologist, Dr. Sumeet K. Mendonca of Ironwood Cancer and Research Centers sent me to Dr. Jennifer Boll, who determined that I required surgery immediately to clean out the infection. She did the surgery the next day, and I woke up with a drain in my chest and a tightly wrapped dressing. Dr. Boll requested that I wrap the dressing as tight as I could tolerate to prevent fluid from building up in the dead space where the tumor had been removed, or it could become infected again.

I had a few setbacks, but we treated them and by the end of November, I was completely healed. Dr. Boll gave me the okay to begin radiation.

I explained to her that I thought my cancer may have resulted from having had too many x-rays and surgeries under fluoroscopy (a form of x-ray used in the operating room), and that if I could avoid it, I really didn't want to be exposed to more radiation.

"If you have a bilateral mastectomy, you won't require radiation."

"What?" I said. "Why didn't anyone tell me that?"

"Someone should have," she said.

"That's what I'm going to do, then. I'm done having kids. I don't need my breasts anymore. How soon can we get it done?" I asked.

"I won't schedule you until you discuss everything with your husband. Call my office once you've decided."

"I'll call you in the morning."

"If you decide to move forward, I'll get in touch with Dr. Stephanie Byrum. We'd both be involved."

That was a tough evening. Rod and I had so much to discuss, and though I wanted his input, it was ultimately my call. I decided to go ahead with the bilateral mastectomy, and Rod supported me.

But I kept second guessing myself and couldn't sleep. Wasn't this kind of drastic? Would I still feel like a woman without my own breasts? How would I look? I asked myself all the questions women facing mastectomy ask themselves over and over again. It was well after midnight before I finally drifted off. By three in the morning, though, I woke up again. My mind was restless, my thoughts scattered. My brain played Russian roulette as I tried to figure out what was important and what didn't matter. Questions always questions. Rod tenderly stroked my arm while I tossed and turned. His soft touch gave me some comfort, but few answers.

I called Dr. Boll's office in the morning and told her that we had chosen bilateral mastectomy. December 9, 2009, was the date of my surgery.

The days leading up to the surgery were difficult. I knew that the only choice I had was to go through with the surgery, yet the reality was tough to swallow. More surgery! I had thought I would be done with surgery once my legs had healed. Fifty-three surgeries were enough! It didn't seem fair, but I, more than anyone game, knew that life was rarely fair. All the x-rays I had on my legs had likely saved them, but they also had likely given me breast cancer.

I woke up knowing that December 8 was the day that Dr. Boll would draw on my chest with a marker so that Dr. Byrum knew where to cut.

Rod had a softball game, so he wouldn't be able to go with me. I didn't feel like going alone, but it looked like I had to. Sarah was at school. I was on my own. I kept myself busy, so I didn't have to think about it, but I thought about it anyway. Once Rod left for the game, I broke down and cried so long and so hard my eyes were red and swollen. All I could think about was more disfigurement and more pain.

I sat at the kitchen table, deep in thought, when I spotted something moving in the brush outside. On this morning, like so many other mornings, I tried to spot him—my coyote. He blended in with the brown brush and was hard to locate. He was slender and tall and often accompanied by two females. There he was, alone that morning, moving slowly through the brush to find his next meal. I left the table to watch from my living room doors. He was crafty and intelligent and displayed a sense of authority as he moved around the saguaro to survey his surroundings. At night I heard the cries of the pack. Native Americans believed coyotes to be mythological representations of good luck and adaptability. *I could use both of those*, I thought. My heart raced faster in witness to one of God's wild creatures.

Then suddenly, he disappeared into the desert, and the side door opened. "Sarah, is that you?" I hollered,

"Yep," she answered.

"Oh, Sarah, I'm so happy you came. I'm having a tough morning!" I looked toward the door, expecting to see her by herself, but two people stood there, one of them my girlfriend Kelly.

"Oh my God!" I sobbed, falling to the floor. If there was ever a time I needed a friend, this was it. It took me awhile before I could talk. "How'd you pull this one off?" I said as I got onto my knees, then awkwardly, stood up. Kelly hugged me and held on.

"We planned it once you set up the operation," Sarah explained. "It was hard to keep secret. I almost told you plenty of times, but I caught myself." Sarah gave me a hug as soon as Kelly let me out of her embrace. "Did you eat yet, Mom?"

"No, I wasn't hungry, but I am now!"

"Okay, good. Why don't we get a bite to eat at the mall before your appointment?"

The twenty-minute drive to the mall seemed to take five minutes. We chatted about everything and nothing. I couldn't help smiling from the back seat, where I sat because Kelly gets car sick. "I still can't believe you two surprised me! Does Dad know?"

"Of course he does. That's why he went to softball. He knew you'd be in good hands."

"And I thought nobody loved me anymore." I pretended to pout.

"We've got your back, Mom."

Sarah parked her BMW at the side entrance to Dillard's Department store. Like three mischievous kids playing hooky, we giggled as we made our way to the food court for a lunch of French fries and other comfort food. Then we shopped and laughed and cried until it was time for the appointment.

We paid at the last register. I walked briskly and nervously ahead of Sarah and Kelly towards the car, now ready to get this over with. I turned back to the other two, and saw that Kelly was still swinging an in-store shopping bag she was supposed to leave behind. Given the tension of the morning, it struck me as one of the funniest things I had ever seen, and I burst into laughter, a laughter so strong my bladder couldn't withstand it. I peed myself right there in the parking lot.

No longer stressing about the appointment, I could think of only one solution. I sat in the back seat on the way to the plastic surgeon's office, nude from the waist down, my pants and underwear flapping in the breeze outside my window. Having my breasts marked up was no longer the most embarrassing thing that would happen to me that day.

CHAPTER 34

SURGERY RESUMED

Surgery was bright and early in the morning. Dr. Byrum was the breast surgeon and Dr. Boll the plastic surgeon. After the mastectomy was completed, two large metal expanders were placed in my chest in preparation for implants. Drains were also inserted under my armpits to remove fluid from the surgical site. When I woke up, I was in pain, but it was nowhere near as intense as the bone pain I had been used to.

In the weeks following, Dr. Boll injected sterile saline into the access port of the expanders once or twice a week to create space for the gel implants. I chose a size somewhere between a C and D cup, expanded from my natural B cup. Go big or go home.

At some visits, Dr. Boll injected 50cc, but most of the time, I requested 100cc, so I could get the implants more quickly. That was the maximum dose and after getting that much, the pain level intensified dramatically. Sometimes it felt like an elephant was sitting on my chest. Other times I'd experience spasms of the small muscles between the ribcage, and they could be painful as well, requiring a muscle relaxant to alleviate them. Most weeks, I received two fills.

Kelly stayed and helped out for almost a week before flying back to Pennsylvania. I put up a good front for her, but once she left, my self-esteem fell to an all-time low. I was just so tired of surgeries and pain and disfigurement. And despite what the doctors told me about the success of these operations, I thought I was going to die. In fact, I was convinced of it.

I had lost so much weight I looked skeletal. I sorted through my clothing to determine what to keep and what to give away and to whom. *I might as well give it all away. Where I'm going, I won't need it.* I asked Sarah what she wanted, but she was aghast. "Mom, no, I don't want your stuff. You need it." I gave the larger clothing and shoes to friends, telling them I was cleaning out my closets and to donate the clothes if they couldn't use them. I even gave away a full-length mink coat (which really upset Rod when he found out years later). When I gave away my jewelry, Sarah took some this time as did my friends. No one suspected what was really going on. Remember, I'm a people pleaser, practiced in pretending to be happy. I just didn't think I was going to beat this one.

Dr. Boll had me wrap myself snuggly in the dressing to avoid the problems of infection due to the fluid buildup. She kept the drains in for ten days, until the drainage was minimal. When the dressing got too tight, Dr. Boll told me, I should remove the dressing and before I put it back on, I should examine the incisions to make sure they weren't infected.

I cried every time I saw the gashes where my breasts used to be. I no longer felt feminine. I no longer felt human. I felt like a medical cadaver, a mad scientist's experiment, a patched together Frankenstein's monster brought to life again and again. I wouldn't let anyone in the bathroom when I was doing this. *It isn't fair. It just isn't fair*, I screamed in my head over and over. I was tired and depressed, and I wanted it all to end. Endless suffering changes a person.

I was going for the big boob look, but the expansion was becoming more painful with each fluid injection.

When the expansion was complete, I had to wait six months before having the surgery to remove the expanders and replace them with gel implants. After the implant surgery, we were concerned with the bluish color and cold temperature of both breasts. Dr. Boll explained that it meant the implants were likely too large. She recommended smaller implants, which meant more surgery. In the next few years, I had surgery three more times to insert smaller implants in hopes of improving the circulation to my chest wall. None of the surgeries were successful, and I developed infections inside my chest twice, requiring additional surgeries to clear the infection.

Since those surgeries weren't working, Dr. Boll proposed another kind of surgery called fat-graft transfer surgery, which she hoped would improve my circulation before my chest tissue became necrotic. With this surgery she harvested fat from various places on my body, then, one drop at a time, placed the fat into my chest cavity to form a boob. She said it would take a minimum of five such surgeries to accomplish. She was right. The temperature and color of my chest didn't improve until after the fifth fat-graft transfer—a long, slow slog. We had to wait six months between surgeries, which were very lengthy with many hours of anesthesia, after which I'd experience extreme nausea and vomiting for days. I had to wear compression undergarments for months afterwards, garments that were hot and tight and not fun to wear in the summer.

Over time, my mental state improved, but then I'd experience lengthy intermittent bouts of depression even the psychiatrists didn't know how to treat. They tried many antidepressants without success. One day I'd wake up depressed without cause and then weeks later, it would resolve as quickly as it had come on. I became so depressed I wouldn't leave the house for weeks, barely talking or eating, let alone doing anything remotely productive. I stopped talking to all my friends until the depression lifted. My family struggled with my depression as well, trying without success to coax me out of it. The depression was all consuming. No one really understood it, including myself.

Then on top of all that, one day I was struck by an intense abdominal pain, extreme nausea, and vomiting without any apparent cause. Several tests confirmed I needed my gall bladder removed. I had the surgery but remained sick. This was at the beginning of the summer, so as soon as I received medical clearance, we headed east to our beach house. We probably should have waited. The trip was a misery, the nausea and vomiting continuing unabated. At one point, I asked Rod to roll me out of the RV into the roadside ditch and leave me for dead. I wasn't kidding. I felt that awful! It took weeks before everything returned to anything resembling normal.

....

CHAPTER 35

FALSE HEART ATTACK

The summer of 2014 started like most summers at the Jersey Shore. Rod and I drove our forty-five-foot RV across the country and arrived before Sarah, who was flying in. We had patio furniture to put outside and spring flowers to plant. The swimming pool had already been opened, but there was always much to do inside the house after being away for seven months.

My girlfriend Kelly and her family were renting the house next door and would arrive in a few weeks, but first Carole, Lindsay, and Eric visited from Connecticut. We always had fun together at the Jersey Shore—long, lazy days on the beach followed by cookouts and clambakes; trips to neighboring islands for shopping and sightseeing; and when we really got bored, there was New York City. We had been coming to Wildwood for years, so we knew the best places to get coffee and pastries, seafood, and Italian food and pizza.

One afternoon, while on the beach, Rod, Carole, and I headed home a bit early. It was unusually hot, and I wasn't feeling quite right. My chest was tighter than usual, but I didn't want to tell the others and spoil their day. After getting out of the shower, the pressure on the left side of my chest increased tremendously, and nothing I did to relieve it—deep breathing, changing positions, stretching—seemed to work. Even with all the pain I had gone through, this was new. I grew short of breath and broke out in a sweat. *Heart attack*, I thought. My father had had his first at forty-two and his father had died of a heart attack in his early fifties. I was fifty-eight.

Rod came upstairs for his shower and saw me pressing my hands to my chest. "What's wrong?"

"A weird chest pain," I said. "I hope it's not a heart attack!"

"Are you serious? What should I do?"

"Roll me a joint, please?" I had been using medical marijuana since it had become legal in Arizona in 2012 to manage pain, symptoms of PTSD, and to relieve anxiety. I was leery at first because I was in recovery, but one of my doctors recommended it to relieve the excruciating pain I felt at night. It had been a great help to me.

I walked into our closet to get dressed and collapsed on the floor. "Hurry," I hollered from the floor. "It's getting worse."

He entered the room holding the unlit joint. "Should I call an ambulance?"

"No. Just light the joint and give it to me." I clamped my eyes shut against the tears of pain.

I accepted the lit joint and took a long drag, then smoked it down to nothing, opening my eyes only to flick the ashes away. But the pain was worsening. I also felt my heart fluttering and my pulse weakening. The nurse in me grew concerned.

"Roll me another one," I hissed against the pain.

"I should call 911."

"Let's try one more. If this doesn't work, we'll call."

I blindly extended my hand for the new joint.

I smoked that one even more quickly than the first. Adrenalin pumped through my body, but the relief I was hoping for never took hold. My heart was now jumping like a vibrating desk toy. I gripped my chest even more tightly, "You better call 911," I told Rod. "Tell them I'm having chest pains! I'll wait in the living room. And could you please tell Carole?"

I took the elevator down to the living room and lay on the sofa. I was hyperventilating without even knowing it, and my fingertips went numb from the shallow breathing. When we heard the ambulance, I went on the porch and sat in the wicker chair while Rod directed the ambulance crew.

The crew rushed to my side. I gave them a detailed medical history, including that of my family. I told them that I had been a critical care nurse and that I was having premature heart beats. They saw I was right when they hooked me up to the heart monitor. They put an IV in my arm then loaded me into the ambulance. Since the kids were still on the beach, Rod was going to wait for them. Carole rode along with me in the ambulance. We stopped two blocks from the house. "Picking up another paramedic," one of them explained. *Oh, great*, I thought. *This crew doesn't know what it's doing.*

In the trauma room at the hospital, two doctors and many nurses went to work, some asking questions, others performing tasks. They did an EKG and blood work and gave me oxygen through a nasal canula.

A short time later, the doctor returned with the EKG results and preliminary lab reports. He didn't think it was a heart attack. He thought the pain was caused by muscles spasms between my ribs, but he admitted me to the hospital, so they could run more tests. "You're also hyperventilating. A nurse will bring you a paper bag to slow your breathing down."

I was given an injection of Toradol and a paper bag and within a short time the pain eased. It felt wonderful to breathe again. That's when the two joints caught up to me. *About time*, I thought, enjoying the bubble of euphoria. I didn't realize how high I was. By the time Sarah and Lindsay arrived, I was briskly tapping away on the sides of the litter, sending messages to the nurses at the desk with the special code we used in circumstances like this.

"Mom, what are you doing?" Sarah asked when she came in the room.

"Sending messages to the nurses out there."

"What are you talking about?"

"I helped them figure out that the guy who came in after me had a heart attack."

"No, Mom. You didn't do that!"

"Sure, I did. I'm using the tapping language I learned in nursing school." I demonstrated by tapping on the siderail. "I just told them the man in bed one just had a heart attack, which his elevated CPK enzymes confirms. They know what I'm saying."

"Mom smoked two joints before she left the house," Rod explained.

"Argh," Sarah said in exasperation. "Mom, please stop it right now. That's embarrassing! You'll be in your room soon. Try to rest quietly."

Fine, I huffed. *I'm just trying to help.* But I stopped tapping.

After a long nap, I woke up, mortified when I remembered the tapping. Thank God the nurses had no clue how stoned I had been. That evening I said to Sarah, "What the hell was I thinking?"

"Not a whole heck of a lot," Sarah replied. "You were stoned out of your mind."

"At least you have some good stories to tell."

"You have no idea!"

The next morning I was told the extra tests showed that the more specific cardiac enzymes were negative for a heart attack. I was discharged later that morning with a prescription for muscle relaxants. *Thank the Lord for small miracles!*

+ + +

This was just one of many medical procedures I endured in the years after the breast surgery.

Due to the overuse of my hands and wrists on my wheelchairs, I needed carpal tunnel surgery on both wrists in 2010. This surgery wasn't too bad pain wise, but it was pretty tough to have my hand in an immobilizer until it healed. Then I did it again nine months later.

When my white blood cells suddenly dropped without explanation in 2011, doctors decided to complete a bone marrow aspiration to make sure I hadn't developed a blood disease. The marrow was harvested from my spine under general anesthesia. The results were negative, but waiting for the results seemed to take forever.

I also had a complete and a partial tear of my left rotator cuff. That was a tough surgery because my left arm remained immobilized for six weeks after surgery in 2021. Rod had to help me dress, as well as blow dry my hair with a round brush. It was pretty funny to watch him try! It was also funny to watch him take my hair in his fist and try to make a big ponytail on top of my head before bed.

I also had progressive neurological damage to some of my toes on both feet due to the limb-lengthening procedure. Five toes developed hammer toe deformities and had to have the distal joints removed to allow them to return to a flat position. This was done in 2022. I could finally wear closed-toe shoes without tremendous pain.

It seemed as if one thing after the next kept occurring. Emotionally I was drained. The continual pain was wearing me down. I kept waiting for the other shoe to drop. Would the next thing be the one that killed me? I worried. Then I worried that it wouldn't be. I grew obsessed with the cancer returning. I'm not typically a worrier, but I worried so much about the cancer returning I gave myself a stomach ulcer. I took medicine for the ulcer and eventually it healed, but only after months.

In total over the thirteen years after I was diagnosed with breast cancer, I required forty-two other surgeries. Since the accident, I had had ninety-three surgeries. Before the accident, I had had nine surgeries. I've now had 102 surgeries in my life! I pray that that's it. No more surgeries!

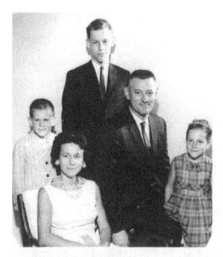

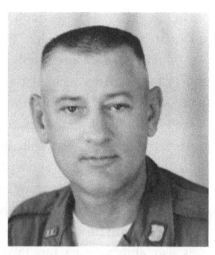

Baur Family Picture, 1962. L to R back row: Kevin (8 yrs.) and Kenneth (15 yrs.); front row: Marion, Charles, and me (6 yrs.).

My father, Charles K. Baur, U.S. Army, Chief Warrant Officer, approximately 1964.

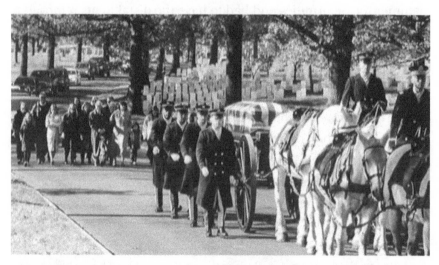

Funeral procession for my father, Charles K. Baur, at Arlington National Cemetery, Arlington, Virginia, November 2016. A rank honored funeral included "Full Military Honors," which meant a caisson escort with military pallbearers marching to the gravesite, a firing party, bugler, folding of and presentation of the U.S. Flag, and a military marching band. My father was predeceased by my mother, Marion S. Baur, and my father-in-law, John R. Shipe, who is buried several rows away. My husband's father, John, was a Full Bird Colonel in the U.S. Air Force.

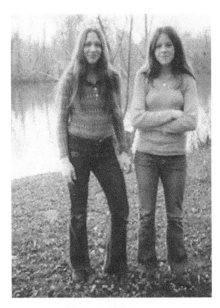

Me and my friend, Shelley J. Kitchura, standing in front of Angelica Dam at the Angelica Park, Reading, Pennsylvania, 1970. Shelley worked with me for four years during the beginning stages of writing my book.

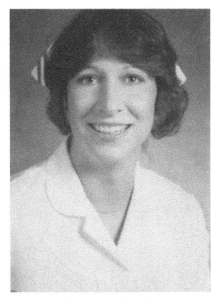

Graduation from Reading Area Community College as a Registered Nurse, May 1983.

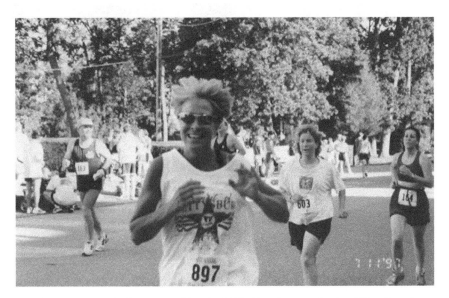

I had been a runner before my accident in 2002. Here I am running in a 5K at Gettysburg National Park, Gettysburg, Pennsylvania, July 1997.

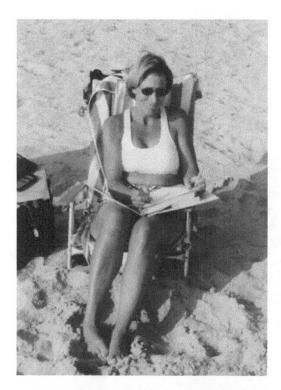

My attorney had this picture of me professionally mounted and displayed in court as a 2' x 3' color image to prove my legs weren't injured before the 2002 accident. I'm sitting on Diamond Beach, New Jersey, working on a child safety program for the Gainfield Elementary School in 1999.

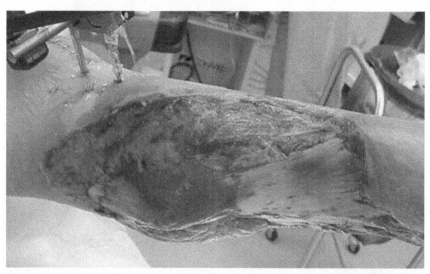

The back of my left lower leg, photographed after I was under anesthesia in the operating room, May 2002. I had lost 90 percent of my calf muscle. The light section is my tendon. Muscles do not have a good enough surface blood supply, so a wound vac was placed over the remaining calf muscle to establish a blood supply, enabling the skin grafts to survive in future surgeries.

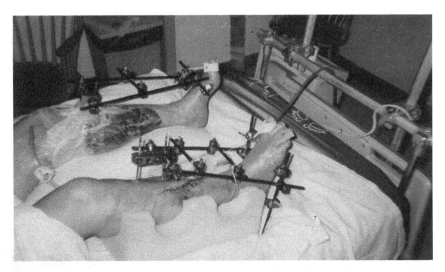

I woke up the morning after the accident with these surgically-placed fixators intact, stabilizing all my fractures. Once the fractures healed, new fixators were surgically placed for limb-lengthening to occur. Two toes on my right foot also had pins sticking out of them. A large charcoal filter covering my left lower leg is the wound-vac system used to establish a better blood supply before skin grafting surgeries could occur.

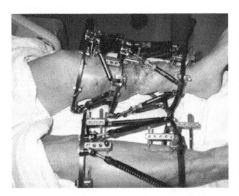

Bilateral lower legs kept intact with Taylor Spatial Frames (all frames are known as "fixators"). My right leg is bolted into a single frame. My left leg is more complexly bolted with a double ring configuration. Dr. Dror Paley, world renowned limb-lengthening expert, initially cared for me at Sinai Hospital in Baltimore. He is now the Director of Paley Orthopedic & Spine Institute at St. Mary's Medical Center, West Palm Beach, Florida.

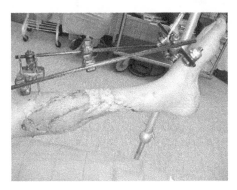

My left lower leg with several successful skin grafts seen over what was raw flesh. Photographed while I was under general anesthesia in the operating room, mid-June 2002. The dotted-Swiss pattern results from the thin slice of skin being removed from my upper thigh, then doubled in length and width by putting it through a machine that punches holes in the skin, creating the ability to cover a larger surface area. Near my ankle is a piece of impregnated gauze used to keep the graft site moist.

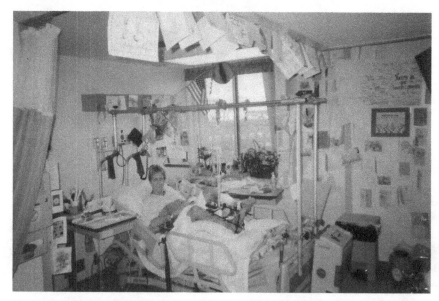

My first hospital room at Yale. Rod, my kids, and Heather hung all the supportive cards and pictures from family and friends.

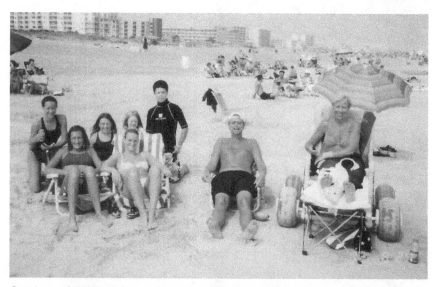

On Diamond Beach at the southern tip of Wildwood, New Jersey, August, 2003.
L to R behind: Jenny (Knoebel) Subers, Maggie Lacon, Claire Lacon, Dan Lacon. L to R front: Sarah (Shipe) Pouncey, Megan (MacKenzie) Panico, MD (my physical therapist at Yale and now a doctor), Rod Shipe, and me on one of two chairs with special wheels that we could borrow from the Wildwood Crest Lifeguards. Eventually, we got our own golf car with oversized wheels.

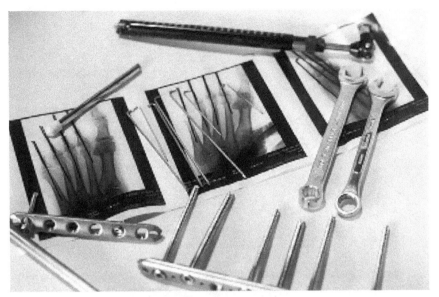

A collection of hardware I've kept over many years and dozens of surgeries.
Left top of frame: A pin that broke off of the Taylor Spatial Frame on my left lower leg.
Right top: Wrenches used to tighten blots on the Taylor Spatial Frames as well as a broken strut at the uppermost part of the picture. Color-coded rings show on the top of each strut, with typically six struts per frame. A computer-generated schedule indicated where I was to turn each color-coded strut daily, an extremely painful process but the only way to regrow bone.
X-rays: My left foot in three different positions showing two pins intact in each of the four toes, after a severe hammertoe deformity was corrected in 2021. The deformity occurred due to nerve damage resulting from the limb lengthening. The pins are sitting on top of the x-rays.
Left foreground: The metal crank I used to turn the Lizarov Device to regrow bone—a painful process of daily breaking the uppermost bone so that new bone would be pulled down and established.
Right foreground just above the crank: Two pieces of titanium hardware and screws that were attached to my left tibia and fibula. I decided not to keep the largest plate and screws.

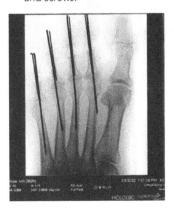

Recent x-rays from March 2021 of my left foot with pins intact after a toe surgery to help correct the progressive neurological toe damage that occurred because of the limb-lengthening ordeal I went through in 2004. These 8 pins remained intact for six weeks until full fusion occurred. Then, without me being on any anesthesia, the PA used pliers to pull two pins out at a time from each toe. Ouch! That hurt. Then I was placed in a soft cast another 4 weeks until my toes healed completely.

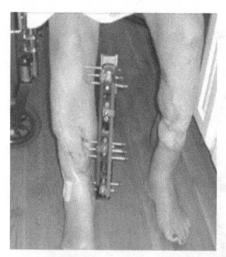

In this picture, a Lizarov External Fixator is attached to my right lower leg bones. This device was surgically placed at Yale by Dr. James Yue. Despite the great pain, I had to turn a crank on the Lizarov each day to break my bone and grow the 7cm of bone to replace the bone that got pulverized in the accident.

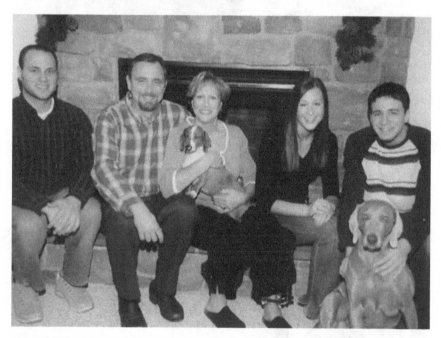

Shipe Family Christmas Picture at home in Sinking Spring, Pennsylvania. L to R: Jason, Rod, me (holding Riley), Sarah, and Adam with Madison, our Weimaraner, 2004. You can see fixators showing below my pant legs.

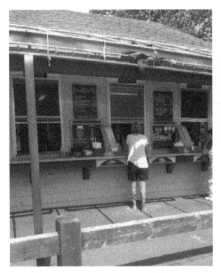
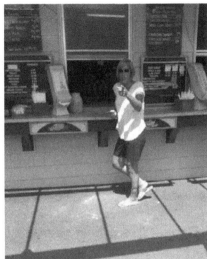

On July 27, 2013, nine years after the accident, I returned to stand in front of Denmo's Take-Out Restaurant in Southbury Connecticut, to tell Dennis, the owner, that I'd forgiven him for not having proper barriers in front of his restaurant. The wooden rails are new.

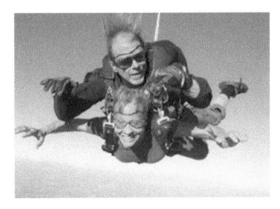

My first skydiving jump with John, a tandem instructor from Skydive Arizona in Eloy, Arizona, March 2018.

PART V

....

THE ROAD
TO HEALING

FAITH, FORGIVENESS, FUN
(AND LOTS OF THERAPY)

The most beautiful people are those who have known
defeat, known suffering, known struggle, known loss,
and have found their way out of the depts. These
persons have an appreciation, a sensitivity, and an
understanding of life that fills them with compassion,
gentleness, and a deep loving concern. Beautiful
People do not just happen.[7]

—*Elizabeth Kubler-Ross, MD*

CHAPTER 36

HAPPINESS IS A CHOICE

I don't want to give the impression that what I've been through was easy. It was not. Before the accident, the worst pain I had experienced was labor. The pain in my legs was orders of magnitude worse than labor, and I pray that you never understand and that you never have to experience that kind of pain yourself.

Pain medication helped, but it didn't eradicate the pain, it just took the edge off, merely allowed me to live with the pain. It was also very difficult to deal with the disfigurement of my legs, my left arm, my chest. I had one setback after the next. I truly seemed to be the unluckiest patient in history.

It took me a long time to accept the fact that healing was going to take many years, and that even when I healed, I wouldn't be the same person I was before the accident. Would I ever feel feminine again? Would I ever be able to work as a registered nurse? Would I ever be able to run? Would I ever feel like a contributing member of society? I had so many questions that went unanswered for so many years. No one really knew the answers.

Even in the earliest days in the hospital, I asked the question: "How long is it going to take?" I was thinking weeks, months. I thought my recuperative powers were in direct proportion to how badly I wanted to get better.

No one wanted to answer that question. Sometimes they looked at me with sympathy and compassion, other times with a look that said, "You don't want to know." Finally, Dr. Yue said, "At least one year." *That shows how much he knows*, I scoffed. *I'll do it in half the time.*

But when six months became a year, and a year became two, then three and more, I couldn't handle it. I had set myself up for failure. When I wasn't up and running by my self-defined milestones based on nothing but magical thinking, I fell apart. I became depressed. I wanted to die. It wasn't until I learned to wait patiently—that I learned to let go and let God—that I came even close to accepting my condition. Waiting taught me compassion, gratitude, humility, and trust in God. Waiting taught me how resilient I was, how courageous I could be.

But I learned only in fits and starts. On one of my last visits to Yale, long after we had already relocated to Pennsylvania, I made an appointment to see Dr. Shin, my plastic surgeon. It had been some time since I had seen him. Once in his office, I said, "I know this is premature because I still have fixators on my legs, but when I'm finally finished with all the limb lengthening, can you do surgery to minimize the scars?"

He didn't respond for a bit, then said, somberly, "Kim, you and me and God did our very best with every one of your surgeries. You still have both legs, and we were never sure we could save even one. Now you must learn to love what you have, who you are. There's nothing I can do about the scars. These are your new limbs, scars and all. In eastern medicine we encourage yoga and meditation and maybe these could help you to love your new self."

"Thank you, Dr. Shin," I said quietly, tears welling. I didn't know if he heard me.

Rod pushed my wheelchair out of the office. I was silent until we reached the car in the parking garage, and then I sobbed. "What a heartless bastard. He has no idea how difficult people have made it for me. They joke about the fixators, and I'm sure they'll joke about the scars. I HATE HIM! I HATE HIM! I HATE HIM!"

That was certainly how I felt then. It took me many years before I could admit that Dr. Shin had been right, and that I was happy to have my legs just the way they were; and even more years after that, with lots of persuading by family and friends, before I could wear shorts or a dress in public. The reality is that no one is perfect. I see everyone else's imperfections every day. Why should I hide mine?

As if the legs hadn't been enough, then I had to deal with a bilateral mastectomy, along with new scars and an even more drastically altered body image. I joke that I'm scarred from tits to toes.

Eventually, I attended cancer support group meetings, and my family also encouraged me to seek one-on-one counseling. I was prescribed antidepressants, and I talked with other women who had gone through breast cancer.

One of the most important things I learned from all these ups and downs is that happiness is a choice, a choice I needed to make every day. (Still need to!) I was going to be exactly as happy as I decided to be; the choice was always in my hands! It no longer mattered how many more surgeries I had ahead of me. That was all in the future, and no one could predict the future. And what happened in the past no longer mattered; it had already happened. I needed to live in the present; the present was all I had any control over. Waiting around for an indefinite future—in my case, one in which I was whole and healthy—was wishing time away. I was wishing away precious time with my husband, my children, and my family and friends. In the end, time is all we have!

My time was all I had, and my time had been filled with trauma. But here's the thing. Each trauma made me stronger. Every time I got stronger I was better equipped to deal with the next hardship. By the time the accident occurred, I was already incredibly strong, and I knew I'd survive. All that adversity saved my life, a profound insight. I wasn't a victim—I was the champion, on top of the world.

Emotionally, however, I struggled for quite some time. I tried to not burden my husband and children with too much because they had their own issues to deal with related to the accident. Picture a stone skipping across a pond and creating ripples every time it slaps the water. I was the stone and my family was the pond. Each time I hit the water, I sent out ripples that affected everyone. Every time I had another surgery or a setback from a previous one, every time they saw the unimaginable pain I was in, they experienced the pain and trauma with me. Meanwhile, all the attention was on me. They were the forgotten sufferers.

Having witnessed the accident and the aftermath, Adam and Sarah both developed PTSD. Rod also developed PTSD because of his relentless vigil at my bedside—twenty-four hours a day, seven days a week, for three-and-a-half months as he watched me suffer beyond belief and advocated on my behalf.

As a result, we've all had counseling and three of us required antidepressants. One of the children became a cutter—slashing their forearms with a razor or knife to punish themselves for the accident, thinking that if they hadn't been fighting, I wouldn't have been standing in front of Denmo's at just that time, and I wouldn't have been hit by the car. Once we found out, we got them professional help and the behavior ended immediately. Although a mother's love can be a potent thing, I soon learned that some things were out of my control, that I couldn't heal anyone but myself.

Rod told me about an interesting exchange in one of his first counseling sessions after the accident. Apparently, Rod referred to me in the past tense when he spoke about me with the counselor. Out of sympathy and to get his background straight in order to help him, the counselor asked him when I had died. At first, Rod was confused. Why would she ask such a silly question? When she explained that he kept referring to me in the past tense, he said he didn't know he was doing that. This gave him pause. On an unconscious level, I had already died to him. He felt guilty about that and apologized profusely. But at one level, he was right. The old Kim had died in the accident, something he—something we all—needed to come to terms with.

In response to my many illnesses and surgeries, Rod also developed a form of what used to be called Munchausen Syndrome. Now it's called *factitious disorder*.[8] Someone with factitious disorder either fakes an illness or injury or induces one in order to bring attention on themselves. I didn't even know it was happening until my girlfriends pointed it out. When I paid attention, I saw the patterns. Whenever I had a big surgery or procedure coming up, Rod would come down with some kind of illness or another—a bad cold, the man flu, a sprained ankle or wrist, a pulled muscle in his back—and he'd want me to take care of him. I usually did. I'm a people pleaser, and my mother had taught me and my brother to wait on my father to keep him calm because of his heart (and his drinking). Rod must have seen that in me. He believed in traditional male and female roles and had been doted on by his grandmother—and wanted me to do the same. Because everything revolved around me for so long after the accident and breast cancer, he faked or exaggerated illnesses to get my attention and the attention of others. And because I'm a people pleaser, I never really called him out on it. Now that I'm healthier myself, he's not ill as often either, though during a recent bout of Covid, he never left the couch, even though the rest of us who got it went about our daily routines without much of an interruption.

We all healed at our own pace. Some of us were willing to work harder while others felt like no one really understood—no one really *could* understand, because they hadn't witnessed such a horrific, catastrophic, life-changing event themselves. We also moved several times after the accident, and as a result, there was little continuity of therapy. As a mom and nurse, I wish I could have fixed all four of us with the snap of my fingers, but that's not how it works. I am aware of my limitations. I can only offer suggestions and information, and the rest is between them and the Lord.

I don't know what I would have done without my extended family and friends. They listened to me and offered advice. Sometimes I just needed to cry, and they were there to pick me up.

I have been seeing the same therapist for quite a few years now. I have shared so much with Dr. Libby Howell that she seems more like a good friend than a therapist. She has given me great advice, always offering solutions in her calm and nonjudgmental way. Libby is also certified in Somatic Experiencing Therapy. At one point, several years into therapy, she asked me if I wanted to try it. She encouraged me to read the book, *Waking the Tiger*, by therapist and author, Peter Levine, in which he describes the use of somatic experiencing therapy to heal trauma.[9]

Dr. Levine's theory (much simplified) is that, when a person undergoes some form of trauma, such as an accident or sexual assault, their body becomes locked in flight, fight, or freeze mode and feels as if it is always under attack. By various exercises, such as mindfulness and deep breathing, somatic experiencing therapy releases the body from the flight, fight, or freeze mode, allowing it to return to a restful healing mode.

I knew immediately I wanted to give it a try.

After my accident, I found it to be extremely difficult to describe to others what happened that day. The images of my mangled, dangling legs when I saw them for the first time are forever imprinted in my memory. When I tried to describe the details again, for example to Officer Don in the hospital when I was giving my statement, I felt as if I was experiencing it all over again—the sights and sounds, being pressed against the building, falling back onto the hood of the car. My whole body shook as if I was freezing. At the time it was a mystery. The next time I discussed the accident, the uncontrollable trembling returned. That's when I realized the trembling was related to the trauma. Over time, the trembling grew less severe and eventually went away, but I continued to have nightmares and anxiety attacks.

Dr. Howell introduced me to somatic experiencing therapy about a decade after the accident. When we did the exercises, the trembling resumed. My body was still stuck in the trauma, and certain triggers made me reexperience it. As the therapy continued, the trauma was released little by little and after about two years, the trembling stopped. I no longer felt all this crazy pent-up anxiety. I felt as if I was on my way to being whole again.

I wished so long to be healed, but I had to learn that healing would take time. I had to give up needing to know when that would be. It was a real blessing to realize that I would be healed, just not now. It freed me up to get on with life. I no longer needed to feel powerless over my life because I wasn't waiting for life to happen some other time. I realized that time is too precious. I didn't want to wish any more of it away. I thought about it this way: if I jumped ahead five, ten, fifteen years to when I finally was healed—and there were no guarantees that that would even happen—would my parents be alive? Would our children still be living with us, or would they be married and living far away? Would my friendships still be strong? This way of thinking about things turned me to the present, helped me cherish where I was *this moment* despite my circumstances.

Self-pity is dangerous but oh so tempting, and I struggled to avoid it, especially in the early months of my recovery. One summer day Rod persuaded me to go in my wheelchair to the Wildwood Boardwalk. I agreed, but I was grumpy and anxious. At the time I still had external fixators on both legs, which were elevated in the wheelchair. I was terrified that some inattentive clod would smack into me and undo months of operations and recovery.

As soon as we arrived, I noticed a man in front of me on crutches. For a moment, I empathized with his predicament. Then human nature took over, and I thought to myself, *Damn I wish I was him, not me.* After all, I was in a wheelchair, and he was able to get around on crutches. I looked away, feeling sorry for myself. When I lifted my head again, I didn't see the man with crutches, but I did see a much younger man coming towards me all alone in a motorized wheelchair. A quadriplegic, his limbs were atrophied and immobile, but that didn't faze him. He was blowing into a stiff plastic tube to keep the chair moving. He was managing all by himself on the Wildwood Boardwalk! He wasn't letting his disability define him.

Okay, God. Good one. I get it. I'll never ask to switch places with anyone again, or wallow in self-pity. I am exactly where You want me to be, and I will heal in Your time, not mine!

I obviously had some lessons left to learn.

....

CHAPTER 37

FAITH: LET GO AND LET GOD

There were three people in my life I had to forgive for me to heal, both emotionally and physically. Well, four people, really, to be truthful. My rapist, Brent; my first husband, Dennis; the man who caused the accident, David Cassidy; and me, the hardest to forgive of all.

And how did I forgive? One simple word: Faith.

I don't know how people go through life without faith in the Lord. My faith is essential to me, and I established this foundation as a child. Mom made sure that we went to church, that we were baptized and confirmed, and that we prayed before each meal and at bedtime. She read Bible stories to us from a children's book. By example and with gentle words, Mom taught me how to bring people together and accept one another. She always rooted for the underdog and accepted everyone just as they were.

But it didn't stop there. Once I was an adult, Mom made sure I went to church no matter where we moved. She was always asking, "Did you go to church on Sunday?" It was very important to her that I kept my faith strong.

As soon as I was no longer confined to bed after the accident, I participated in a women's small group Bible studies in Connecticut, where I met many nice and smart women who gave me insight into the Word and offered Christian love and acceptance. I had always longed to read the Bible for a better understanding of my faith, but I had never known where to start.

Once we moved back to Pennsylvania, I grew more confident in my understanding of scripture and led several Bible studies myself at the church we joined. I held the classes in the evenings for both men and women, and they were well attended. I built a strong connection to my faith at the time, which kept me going, since I was still using a wheelchair and desperately needed something outside myself to commit to.

Like many others, though, I sometimes struggled with my faith. It was not that I ever stopped believing, but I experienced times I couldn't pray. I was just too frustrated to ask for yet another thing that wouldn't be granted or relief from pain that wasn't going away anytime soon. I referred to these times as dry spells of faith. At some point, we all find ourselves caught up in a dry spell of faith. That's when it's important to have a connection to a church, a Bible study, or a prayer group, so you can reach out to others to pray for you. My faith community got me through many such times, and I was always grateful for their presence in my life.

At one point, I faced one set back after another. Several of my friends suggested I pray for protection from evil. So I wrote a personal prayer for protection I recited aloud several times a day. It wasn't like a magic spell that worked instantly, but as the days went on, the negativity around me dispersed, replaced by a gladness that filled my heart so that others could see Him and the difference He made in my life. The Lord performs extraordinary acts through the most broken creatures, like me. A diamond is a small chunk of coal that does well under pressure. I prayed that I could be a chunk of coal that becomes a diamond.

Further, I learned to thank the Lord for what He was doing in my life. Sometimes we forget to say thank you because we're already thinking up our next request. We have to remember that God is not our personal vending machine. We must trust in Him, for He gives us what He deems necessary. I often prayed to surrender my pride in exchange for His gift of grace and mercy.

My mom's favorite Bible verse was the Twenty-third Psalm: "The LORD is my shepherd, I shall not be in want. He restores my soul. He guides me in paths of righteousness for his name's sake. Even though I walk through the valley of the shadow of death, I will fear no evil, for you are with me; your rod and your staff, they comfort me."

Whenever I recite this psalm, I feel the peace and comfort of my faith in the power of Jesus Christ. For me, the central message is of God's grace in our lives. He leads us to safety and restores our broken-ness. Because, let's face it, we're all broken, and we desperately need His grace! He waits patiently for us to ask for His help.

There were times when I felt so broken that it seemed too diffi-cult to continue. I felt as if I'd never be whole again. I was wrong! I feel more alive today than in all my yesterdays. The Lord wants nothing other than to give us good things, though they might not always be the things we think we want, nor in the timeframe we request. I will never understand the magnitude of His love for me—for all of us—but I gratefully accept it. In my darkest days, I prayed that I would always remember that, even in my sin, He saw my worth. I prayed to also see the worth in all people, to help me love them as only he did, to sacri-fice my needs and desires so that I may help others. Just one person can change the course of the world.

I believe in Jesus Christ and in the power of the Gospel. I believe in the one whose spirit glorified a small village, of whose coming shepherds saw the sign, and for whom there was no room at the inn. I believe in the one whose life changed the course of history, over whom the rulers of the earth had no power. I believe in the One whom the oppressed, the discouraged, the afflicted, the sick, the blind, and the injured gave welcome, and accepted as Lord and Savior. I believe in the One who with love changed the hearts of the proud and with His life showed that it is better to serve than to be served. I believe in peace, which is not the absence of war, but the presence of justice and love among all people and nations. I believe in reconciliation, forgiveness, and the transforming power of the gospel. I believe that I must be the change the world needs to see.

It excites me to know that when I am in the light of God in heaven, my scars will disappear. I will be whole again in his eyes. Even here on earth, God's grace has sustained me. I loved to linger in His presence as I ever so slowly healed. God never gave me more than I could handle; instead, he gave me the tenacity and the will to heal and forgive. He showed me that my accident and cancer did not define who I was. I had lost myself in the morass of medical issues and setbacks. I became a wretched, fractured, cancerous, lifeless being. He took me on a detour and showed me the way back.

We should always look for God's detours—and follow them. It was during some of my life's detours that the Lord gave me hope, gave me peace, gave me the most unexpected joys! My detours slowed me down, taught me what was important. Just as the Lord rested on the seventh day, we need to take time to rest, to dream, to renew our strength. On one of God's detours I realized that I didn't have to carry the burden of shame that a naïve, raped thirteen-year-old had imposed on herself, that it was a spiritual cancer that gnawed at my soul. Faith in Him transformed this most broken spirit and splintered human being.

I have downloaded two applications to my phone to help me focus on faith. One is Holy Bible KJV. At eight in the morning and eight in the evening, a beautiful chime plays to remind me to read a Bible verse, an inspiration, and a prayer. The other is Mission 119, also called 91 weeks with Jesus. Five days a week scripture is read to you and then a pastor interprets the passage for a greater understanding. This morning ritual takes about twenty minutes and if you do this for five days each week, in 91 weeks you will have read the entire Bible. I have already

completed Mission 119 once, and I just started to partic
second time. There's so much to learn.

I've always thought it's important to giveth as well a
I don't know if Mom would have put it quite that way, but I do know
that she always made it her practice to do so.

I received several prayer shawls when I was sick, one after my accident and another from my daughter-in-law, Jacquelyn, after I developed breast cancer. Jacquelyn's was made of soft, pink yarn, and
I brought it with me into dozens of operating rooms.

While knitting the shawl, the giver prays for the recipient, in
essence weaving the prayer into the garment. I found that to be one
of the most beautiful, precious acts of kindness, and I wanted to pay
it forward. Since I knew how to knit, I founded a prayer shawl min-
istry at my church in Robesonia, Pennsylvania. Members who could
knit or crochet joined up. Once the shawls were completed, our pastor
prayed over them. We made over a hundred prayer shawls during the
four years I lived in that community and delivered them to shut-ins,
to those diagnosed with cancer, to a recently paralyzed young man, to
accident victims, to those recovering from surgeries, to those suffering
with depression, to the lonely, and to so many more. We prayed while
we knitted, our faith strengthened with every word.

Armed with faith, you can do anything. Faith has allowed me to
stop living in fear. When fear dictates our lives, the world shrinks until
we can no longer function. Fear robs us. And why do we have fear? We
have fear when we lose faith. When we surrender in faith to the Lord,
on the other hand, we gain peace. I never thought I had the right to
ask, *Why me?* Because truthfully, none of us is special or immune to
hardship or disease or deserving of some special favor from the Lord.
We live in a fallen world. Life isn't always going to be fair, equal, or just.
It is our faith in the Lord that allows us to transcend life's inequities.
For this I am forever grateful.

CHAPTER 38

FORGIVENESS:
THE GIFT YOU GIVE YOURSELF

Without faith, there is no forgiveness, and without forgiveness, there is no healing.

We must learn to forgive so that we can live in peace without resentment, anger, depression, and undue stress. When we withhold forgiveness, we are only harming ourselves, not the other person. It might be the most difficult thing you do, forgiving someone who has grievously wronged you. You're not doing it for them, though. You're doing it for yourself. A huge weight is lifted from us when we forgive. Forgiveness sets us free from the bondage of the past, moves our soul beyond the pain. Forgiveness is especially rewarding when you've withheld it for a long time. The longer you withhold it, the "sicker" you become. I was broken in body and spirit, and for me to heal, I had to forgive.

Ten years after I was raped, I had the courage to discuss it for the first time with Rod, my husband. We had been married for just over a year. He was the *One*, my soulmate, and I trusted him implicitly. He was shocked, but he didn't want to sweep it under the rug. He encouraged me to get counseling.

I found a very good female therapist to work with and I started to see her on a weekly basis. After a full year of therapy, I felt like I had accomplished what I needed to, so I stopped seeing her. What I didn't realize was that I had not forgiven him, Brent, the rapist. I still hated him. That was understandable, I thought, and only natural, considering what he had done to me.

But that hatred held me prisoner for more than fifty years. I had plenty to deal with with the accident and breast cancer, of course, but whenever I dug into what was eating at me, whether with the help of a therapist or in my own hopeless thoughts at two in the morning, it always came back to the rapes. I realized that if I didn't forgive Brent, I would never heal.

It took me fifty-one years, but I finally wrote a letter to my rapist in 2020. I addressed it to him and his wife using my maiden name and had Shelley mail it from Colorado so he wouldn't know where I lived. (I may have been forgiving him, but I certainly didn't want to see him or have him contact me any other way.)

Finally writing this letter was therapeutic, the final step in healing this open wound. I was no longer the scared thirteen-year-old who didn't have the skills to help myself. I forgave him, but I also told him everything I had waited so long to say. I didn't hold back. I called him a rapist, a pervert, a pathetic pig. I told him I hoped he got the help he needed. It was no small satisfaction that he'd likely have some serious explaining to do to his wife.

✦ ✦ ✦

It was easier to forgive David Cassidy, the driver of the car that nearly took my legs. In fact, I forgave him right away.

In the weeks and months after the accident, my pastor visited me often. On one of his visits, he told me that he was also visiting the man who hit me. He asked if there was anything I wanted to say to him.

"Yes, actually, since you asked. Could you please tell him I've forgiven him? I know that no one would have done something like that on purpose. As bad as it was for me, it was an accident."

"That's very generous, Kim," the pastor said, relieved. Who knows what he imagined I would say. "That'll mean a lot to him. He's taking it hard. He feels so guilty for what he's done to you and your family."

After the pastor visited him, David Cassidy sent me a beautiful prayer card with the message that he would pray for me every day for the rest of his life and that he had paid for Catholic masses to be said for me. This was a beautiful and kind gesture. Sometimes prayer is the only thing another person can do for us, and for us believers, prayer is often enough.

What I didn't learn for a long time afterwards, though, was that just a few weeks after we exchanged messages, David passed away from an unexpected heart attack. It was a somber moment when I learned of his death. I knew then I would never meet him, but I was thankful that he knew I had forgiven him before he died. At least he passed on without that burden of guilt.

+ + +

I have another story of forgiveness, now that I think of it.

It was the summer of 2012, and I was invited to Connecticut because my friend Sue was hosting a party. I arrived a few days early so I could help her set up. Everything was going as planned, then our friend, Carole, asked us to meet her at Julio's Restaurant for a few drinks to celebrate her birthday. Sue told me to go in the car along with her friend, David, and she would meet us at the restaurant. I didn't know David well and thought it strange that she wanted me to drive with him.

It turns out that David was easy to talk to, a great listener. The conversation turned to my accident, and for once I didn't mind talking about it. In fact, that was just about all we talked about the whole ride, and we were both very intent on the conversation. (I no longer shook uncontrollably when I talked about it.) When we got to the traffic light on Main Street, instead of turning right toward Julio's, David turned left by accident.

"No, that's the wrong way," I said. "But since we were talking about it, Denmo's is just over there." I gestured toward the right side of the street.

"Do you mind if I drive there?" David said.

"No, that's fine. It's right there." I pointed.

David slowed the car and pulled into the parking lot. "I hope you don't mind."

"I guess not," I said. I'm a very spontaneous person. I just rolled with whatever happened next. I was sure that David meant no harm, and I felt that I could trust him.

"Where were you parked that day?" he asked.

"Right there in that empty space." I pointed. I'm not sure why I answered him. It seemed like the right thing to do.

He inched the car forward until we were parked in the exact space I had parked in just over ten years before. I sat there silently agitated as the memories of that day flooded through me.

"Where were you standing when it happened?"

"I was standing right there at the second window when I ordered our food. The driver was pulling into the parking space directly behind me, except those wooden abutments weren't there ten years ago. All that separated the car from me were some white lines on the asphalt."

"Could we get out of the car and go to the corner of the building before you finish your story?"

I took a deep breath. "I guess so, but it's going to be a little scary!" I opened the door and ever so slowly exited the car. David waited for me and together we walked to the front corner of the building. I could feel my heart racing, and I started to breathe faster. Even though the wooden rails had been installed between the parking lot and the order windows, I didn't think the rails would really stop a car. I stood less than ten feet away from where I had been hit. I was extremely nervous. I scanned the parking lot in a constant motion, scrutinizing every car that pulled in.

"I don't know how long I can stand here," I said.

"We can leave whenever you want to."

"Okay." I rubbed my sweaty palms together and played nervously with my fingers as I have since childhood.

"You said that you were standing at the second window to place your order. Then what happened?"

"Well, the kids' orders were complicated. I was concerned about getting the order correct. When I was sure I got it right, I paid for everything and then put the change in my wallet."

"What were you going to eat yourself that day?" David asked.

"A dish of vanilla ice cream."

"Why don't you and I go to the second window and place an order for the ice cream you never got to enjoy. I'm buying!" David gestured for me to follow him.

I froze in fear, reluctant to move. It was unthinkable, what he was asking me to do, but I knew I should follow his lead to fully heal. Slowly, I walked to the second window. There was someone in front of us, placing their order. I couldn't face the window, but turned instead to watch the traffic, my heart pounding.

"It's our turn. What would you like?" David asked.

I looked at the young girl and said, "A medium dish of vanilla ice cream, please."

David said, "And I'll have a medium dish of seafood ice cream!"

We laughed. I knew David was trying to ease my nerves.

"Actually, I have a story to tell you," I said to the young woman taking our order.

David said, "No, not yet. Wait until we get our ice cream and then you can tell her your story."

"Okay," I said, scanning the parking lot again.

"I'll have the same thing she ordered," he said.

She totaled the order, and David paid for it. When she returned with our ice cream, David said, "Okay, tell her!"

I looked behind me again to make sure it was safe. Then I said, "Ten years ago, I came here with my two children. I ordered food for them and ice cream for myself, but I never got to eat my ice cream. While I was waiting for my order, an elderly man drove into the parking lot and hit me with his car and smashed me into the building. Today David brought me here so I could finally get the ice cream I never got to eat ten years ago."

"Oh my gosh," she said. "Can you tell her?" She pointed to the young girl standing at the first window.

"No, I'm too nervous to stand here any longer. I'm sorry, you'll have to tell her. Thanks for the ice cream!" I walked briskly towards the picnic tables, and when I reached them, I got onto my knees and out loud I said a prayer of gratitude for small miracles. I stood up and said to David, "Do you mind walking behind the restaurant with me? That's where I asked the police to take the kids after the accident so they couldn't see what was happening."

"Not at all," he said.

We walked around the left side of the building and stopped in the back. I remembered it all as if it had happened yesterday.

"Kim is that you?" someone called out, interrupting my thoughts. It was Marilyn, Dennis's wife. They owned Denmo's together.

"Yes, it's me," I said as I walked towards her. "Marilyn. I came back to get the ice cream I never got to eat ten years ago. How are you doing?"

"I'm okay, but Dennis isn't doing so good. He still blames himself."

"I'm sorry to hear that. I'm doing okay. Do you think I could see Dennis before we head back? Maybe if he saw me, he'd feel better."

"He's not here today. He'll be here tomorrow if you can come back in the afternoon."

"Okay, that's what I'll do, but could you keep it a secret? I'd like to surprise him."

"I won't say a word. You look so good. It was so good to see you!"

On the ride to Julio's I said, "I'm sure everyone's going to wonder where we've been. They won't believe it. I'm not sure I believe it."

When we walked into Julio's, many of my friends were already there.

"Where'd you guys go to?" asked Carole.

"You'll never believe it. We took a wrong turn and ended up at Denmo's. But now I think it was supposed to be. I saw Marilyn and ate the ice cream I never got to eat ten years ago."

"Are you serious? What about Dennis?" Carole asked.

"I'm going to see him tomorrow," I said. "And you're coming with me."

"Okay, Boss. If you say we'll be there tomorrow, we'll be there tomorrow!"

The rest of the night was filled with storytelling and laughter, although in my mind I kept thinking about how ironic it was that we ended up at Denmo's. But I also had room to think about how much their family had suffered as well. We had certainly all suffered far too much for far too long.

The following day, just after lunch, Carole and I made our way back to Denmo's. I usually don't remember my dreams, but the previous night I dreamt about being back in the hospital after my accident. It felt different somehow. I wasn't hurt as bad in the dream, and I felt whole again. My scars were gone. It seemed like a sign.

The parking lot wasn't full when we pulled into a space along the side of the building. We got out of the car and walked towards the ordering windows. It seemed more familiar, less scary than it had the day before.

At the window I said, "Hi, could we please have two medium dishes of vanilla ice cream? And could you tell Dennis that someone is here to see him?"

"Sure," she said as she turned to get our ice cream. "Dennis, someone's here to see you."

She handed us our ice cream, and I handed her my cash. Dennis walked up behind her. He didn't seem to recognize me, even though we were face to face. "Hi Dennis. Do you remember me?" I paused. "I'm Kim Shipe."

His expression went from puzzlement to recognition. "Oh, what a nice surprise, Kim. You look great!"

"I stopped here yesterday to get the ice cream I never got to eat ten years ago. Marilyn said you'd be here today. Can we talk privately?"

"I'll be right out."

Carole and I walked around the back of the building. As soon as I met up with Dennis, I gave him a big hug, which surprised him. I introduced Carole, and after some small talk and ice cream eating, I told Dennis that Marilyn had told me he wasn't doing well since the accident. And then I said, "Dennis, I want you to know that I've forgiven you for any responsibility you think you had for my accident. It wasn't your fault. It was an accident. Look how good I'm doing. The last time you saw me I was in a wheelchair, and now I can walk without a limp." I took a few steps for him. "I want you and your family to heal as well."

His eyes showed a mixture of surprise, buried pain, and vulnerability, as if he wanted to believe but thought it might be too good to be true.

We talked for several more minutes before I said goodbye. We hugged again, and this time he put his whole being into it.

As I walked back to Carole's car, a kind of quiet peace arose within me. I felt like everything had come full circle and we could all get on with our healing. Everything happens for a reason. The Lord had had much bigger plans for my trip to Southbury than simply to see friends and go to Sue's party.

+ + +

I thought I was up to date on forgiveness, but as
the first draft of this book, I was struck with an im
forgiven many people who had harmed or viola
given myself for many things, with one huge o...
forgiven myself for the abortion when I was nineteen.

Of all the things I had experienced, this was the one I tried to think about the least, the one that brought me the most shame. I never thought of myself as a prideful person, but shame is the opposite side of the coin of pride. Having an abortion was something that I never in a million years would have imagined I would do. It didn't fit my image of myself as a compassionate and nurturing Christian woman. Pride had blinded me; it kept me from admitting what I had done. And if I couldn't admit it, how could I forgive myself? How could I grieve?

To get on the path of self-forgiveness, I attended a weekend retreat conducted by Rachel's Vineyard, an organization dedicated to helping women and men heal from post-abortion and miscarriage trauma. The shame and grief of such experiences take an emotional toll. These parents seek resolution for their damaged and broken sense of selves.

It was one of the most significant steps I took to heal. What I learned from the retreat was that by withholding forgiveness from myself, I was treating myself worse than I treated the rapist in my life and the abusive husband. If they were worthy of forgiveness, why wasn't I?

The retreat helped me forgive myself, helped me affirm, that, despite the anger, the anguish, the grief, the bitterness, the depression, the hatred, the fear, the blackness, the pain, the violations, the self-destructiveness, the tears of shame, the suffering, the wounds, the chaos, the confusion, the offenses, the silence, the ugliness, the unthinkable, the lies, the human weaknesses, the loneliness, the isolation, the diminished spirit, the heavy-heartedness, and the sorrow I experienced because of the abortion, I WILL BE HEALED!

In this way, I will transform into the most beautiful butterfly, that symbol of rebirth and renewal. I am now truthfully unobstructed, ready, willing, and able to do His eternal work here on earth. God rgave me upon my first sincere request for forgiveness. He always knew how I felt, since He walked alongside me. I heard His gentle whispers in my ear, even when I didn't think He was there, always encouraging me even in despair to keep on going on. Forward, always forward. I remind myself of that often.

I met the most amazing singer and song writer, Michael John Poirier, who played his songs for us at the Memorial Service for our lost children at the conclusion of the retreat. One song, "Kathryn, John and Mary," spoke to me.[10] Michael gave me permission to include it here.

Kathryn, John and Mary

Kathryn, John and Mary, pray for your Mama tonight
It's been a long, hard road-but in her heart she knows
one day she'll see your smiling face,
and gather you in her arms ...

Kathryn, John and Mary pray for your Mama tonight
as she looks up into a starry sky,
she can't help but sing you a lullaby
and she calls you each by name:

If I had known back then what I know right now
you'd be standing before me someway, somehow
My babies, I love you,
but Mama cannot change the past.
I have wondered for years over oceans of tears,
afraid I had lost you forever
But the darkness is ending
And a new light's beginning to shine

Cause I feel you here ... alive again,
helping your Mama to love again
From now until the day I see you-
You'll be in my heart

Kathryn, John and Mary, pray for your Mama tonight
It's been a long, hard road
but in her heart she knows
one day she'll see your smiling faces,
and gather you in her arms ...

Mama hear our words to you: We promise to
pray the whole night through
And kiss you each time we hear you sigh
till the day the Heavens open wide
Then we'll stand together on Heaven's golden shore
In joy we'll sing forever the mercy of the Lord.

We can't change the past, but we can change the present.

CHAPTER 39

I TRY MY HAND AT BUSINESS

After the bilateral mastectomy, I struggled with my self-esteem as do many women. There is something fundamentally barbaric about hacking off your breasts! It's almost too much to take in.

At first, it was extremely difficult to look at my chest, let alone let anyone else see it. I continued to get infections after surgeries and had to diligently examine and clean the incisions and drain sites. I also had to wear an ace bandage wrapped tightly around my chest to keep seromas from forming.

One day in 2010 I was bored—bored with sitting around and bored with the dull hospital bandages they had given me to wrap my chest. The bandages were the same texture and consistency throughout; some parts were too tight and others too loose. And the color—blech! Why couldn't I make my own, with brighter colors and softer fabrics? I could make them more comfortable. I could make them reversible with different colors or patterns on each side.

I had several things going for me: I was a nurse, so I knew what was required. I could sew, so I knew fabric. I had my own sewing machine. I had also been a runner, had an appreciation for wicking fabric, and

I was bored. This would give me something to do and maybe pick up my spirits and self-esteem.

I liked projects, so I prayed and got started immediately.

First, I had to find the fabrics and then sew the prototype. I narrowed my choices to 80 percent nylon and 20 percent spandex. (Most compression garments are constructed with only 8 percent spandex.) One would be the absorbent middle layer. The other would make up the outer layers. There would be three layers in all, and the outer layer need to be able to wick moisture to the middle layer. For that purpose, I applied a finish called Naturexx to increase the wicking potential. All three layers had to offer maximal stretch and compression without the fibers tearing with repeated use. For that purpose, the cloth was manufactured by means of a warp knitting process first invented in the 18th century.

If I used two colors for the outside layers, the dressing would be reversible. I'd put Velcro closures at both ends, and I could impregnate all three layers of fabric with colloidal silver or a similar product to provide anti-microbial protection. If I found that the fabric slipped out of place with wear, I planned to add silicone dots on one side of the bandage.

It was a beautiful sunny day when I left the house, eager to find the perfect fabric. I chose hot pink, lime green, and bright teal for the outer layers and white for the invisible middle layer. As soon as I got home, I laid the fabric on the floor, where I used my cutting mat, roll cutter, and straight edge to cut the fabric into the correct lengths and widths.

By the end of the day, I had sewn my first three bandages. I took off the Ace bandage and replaced it with the hot pink one. I giggled when I saw myself in the full-length closet mirror. The fabric was so soft against my skin and the stretch in the fabric was more effective than the Ace. When I put my blouse on, I felt as if I was wearing fancy lingerie.

For the first few days I switched to a different color each day. It was so much fun. It did lift my spirits! I already felt better, and not only that, but the bandage also compressed my chest more effectively than other dressings.

When I next met with Dr. Boll, I showed her what I had made. She was so impressed she suggested I make some to sell to the public. She wrapped it and unwrapped it, stretched it this way and that. She said I had thought of everything.

On my drive home, I thought about mass producing the bandages. *I've never started a business before*, I thought. *Or run one. Could I do it?* I had a lot to think about.

In the meantime, I sewed bandages for everyone I knew who had breast cancer and was about to have surgery. I made dressings and shipped them far and wide across the country.

There was much to do before I could start the business. It became on-the-job training.

I hired a patent attorney. To apply for a patent, I had to list the product's features, describe the entire manufacturing process, forecast future considerations, and include graphics. I needed a business name and a tax ID number. I needed to design the bandage boxes, and the package insert. I needed to find a fabric supplier, a manufacturer, a printer, and a box company. Before I could even talk to potential vendors, I had to draft a non-disclosure and non-compete letter.

I would begin by manufacturing a small run of dressings for clinical trials, conducted by Dr. Boll, my plastic surgeon, and Dr. Peter Sebastian, a neurologist who also agreed to participate, using patients with sports injuries and lymphedema.

Pete was Rod's best friend in high school, and they had stayed friends afterwards. Initially, I asked Pete to do some research for me, and he agreed. I paid him an hourly rate for his work. When it became time for the clinical trials, I asked him if he wanted to do that as well, and he said yes. At one point, I was running out of money to invest and offered him 10 percent ownership and he agreed. (I also gave Sarah 10 percent ownership and offered the same to Adam, but he declined.)

To get to the point where we were ready to do the clinical trials took over two years. I made hundreds of phone calls and invested much more money than I could have ever imagined.

We settled on a manufacturer, who produced a small test run that met my approval, then produced several hundred bandages for clinical trials. The biggest issue during trials was one I had anticipated—the dressings shifted out of place when the wearer was active. We added silicone dots to one side of the dressing in the next run, and it worked to keep the bandages in place.

I also designed drain pockets, which could be attached or removed from any bandage with Velcro. I made binders out of the same fabric, which could be used to hold gauze pads anywhere on the body after surgery. They were also great for applying ice packs.

We wanted to sell all over the country—and the world—which meant a website, for which I hired a website designer and videographer.

It was so exciting to see my whim of a bandage project grow into a full-fledged business: Miss Daisy Medical, LLC. I still own and operate this business, though three years ago I sold the bandage portion to a larger company with a broader market reach. The bandages I invented are now sold under the name Python Wrap.

Building a business from scratch is a lot of work, believe me, but it's also fun, a great way to get outside of yourself and stay engaged in the world. And if you're engaged in creative work, you're well on your way to healing.

CHAPTER 40

THE JOY OF RUNNING AGAIN

One day many years after my accident and mastectomy I was in Reading, Pennsylvania to take care of business involving my father's estate after he died in 2016. I was planning to stay for the weekend, and I had brought workout clothing and sneakers along. I called my friend Diane. "Hi Diane. If you aren't busy in the morning, I was wondering if you'd like to meet me behind the Shillington Market for a run?"

"Are you serious?" she said with excitement.

"Yes. I'd like to try our old route. I'm not going to promise anything. I'm going to be slow and might have to walk some, but I'm going to give it a try!"

"I'll be right beside you. I never thought we'd run together again. Can't wait."

At nine o'clock the next morning, I had already stretched and eagerly awaited Diane's arrival. It was a beautiful morning, perfect weather, the best of days to test my new legs.

Diane arrived and parked next to my car. "Are you excited?"

"I could barely sleep last night!"

"What do Rod and the kids think?"

"I didn't tell them."

"Why not?"

"They wouldn't want me to do it. But I have to, you know that. Every time I see a runner, I want to get out there. I've never lost that urge."

Diane nodded while she stretched. As a fellow runner, she got it. "Ready?" she asked.

"Yep." I clicked the timer on my watch and slowly got started. It was all new today. I couldn't push off with my left foot because of the Achilles tendon the doctors couldn't reattach properly. It took effort to lift my foot, and I could hear an audible flap every time it hit the black-top. My right leg felt strong in comparison. The first part of the run was flat and easy, so I focused on the breathing and footing as I tried to get both under control.

"Just let me know when you want to stop," she said.

"I will," I gasped. That was all the talking I could manage. The muscles in my legs trembled, but I pushed harder. Then, as in times past, I caught a rhythm, my breathing slowed, and a calm enveloped me. I smelled the spring flowers and felt the air on my face. I was running!

As we rounded the corner and headed downhill, the pounding on my legs increased. It was time to walk. "Sorry, have to stop," I called out.

"I told you I don't care," Diane said, and slowed to a walk beside me.

"Thanks." When we reached the bottom of the hill, we began to run again. For the next forty-five minutes, we continued the route with brief periods of walking. When we had the finish line in sight, I could barely contain my excitement. I increased my pace and crossed the line in tears.

"I DID IT! I JUST RAN OVER THREE MILES WITH THESE LEGS!" I shouted.

"I never thought I'd see this day!" Diane hugged me, and we laughed and cried together. "I'm so proud of you."

"Thanks, Diane. Thanks for being my wingman."

"I wouldn't have missed it for the world!"

I felt renewed as I drove away from the parking lot. Even if I never ran after that, I had done what I thought I would never do again. I wished my orthopedic surgeons and Dr. Paley could have seen me. I wanted to call Rod, Adam, and Sarah and tell them right away, but I also wanted to see their faces when I gave them the news. I decided to wait.

Once back in New Jersey, I waited until dinner. "Guess what I did this morning?" I announced.

"Met Kelly for breakfast," Sarah responded.

"Nope. I went for a run! With Diane. We met behind the market like we used to and ran three miles. I had to walk at times, but I didn't have any pain while I was running. My legs feel great right now. I'm sure tonight they will hurt as usual."

"I can't believe you did that," Rod said, not as enthused as I had hoped. "You could have injured yourself."

"I was careful, and I was ready to stop if it was too much, but I never needed to."

"Well, that's good, Mom. I'm so proud of you," said Sarah.

Rod's expression suggested he wasn't so sure. But I felt good about my decision. Rod loved me, and I loved him, but sometimes you've got to do what you've got to do, no matter whom you risk disappointing—a very hard choice for a people-pleaser like me.

CHAPTER 41

IF YOU CAN'T TAKE WING, TRY A PARACHUTE

I am a positive person. I am spontaneous. I like to have fun and laugh. I have a good sense of humor. All these traits have contributed to my recovery and healing. Even when I was in the ambulance ready to go to the hospital after the accident, I joked with Officer Don. I can still see his face when I asked him to get a to-go bag for the food I had paid for.

I inherited my sense of humor and optimism from my mother. She thoroughly enjoyed life, living every day like it was her last. She always tried to turn negatives into positives. Like her, I don't allow too much to upset me and that's evident in my bubbly personality and spontaneous laughter. I can even find humor in my own mistakes. Why not?

Did I say I was spontaneous? This is how I ended up jumping out of a plane for the first time in my life at the age of sixty-one. This was in 2017.

Rod and I took a motorcycle trip to Eloy, Arizona, with several of his friends, including my friend Sue, who was visiting me from

Connecticut. In the middle of the Sonoran Desert between Phoenix and Tucson, Eloy is the skydiving capital of the United States, perhaps even the world, with its clear days and uninhabited landscape. We thought we'd get out on the open road, have lunch, and watch the sky-divers, from the bleachers.

The center has two main landing fields. That day, Dutch paratroopers were jumping on one of them and recreational divers on the other. Adrenalin pumped through us as we watched the divers step out of the planes and drop through the air, the wind whipping at their equipment, then popping open their chutes and gliding to the ground one after another, running to a stop with the chutes collapsing behind them. In excitement, Sue asked me if I thought that she could jump. "Let's go to the office and ask," I said, my face flushed with excitement. And off we went.

They told her yes, she could jump. She was very excited, but I had my own ideas brewing in my mind as we walked briskly back to Rod and his three friends.

The guys were surprised when we told them.

"Rod, would you mind if I jump as well?"

"Your legs," Rod said. "Is that a good idea?"

"Your motorcycle," I said in return. "Is that a good idea?"

"Point taken," he said. "Just be sure to tell them about your legs. They may not let you go." I could tell that's what he hoped would happen.

"Got it," I said.

In the office, the attendant said there was room on the last flight, and Sue could definitely have a spot. He wasn't sure about me, though, after I showed him my legs and explained the extent of my injuries. He called in his superior to make the call.

When we explained my situation, he asked me two questions. "Can you squat?"

"Yes," I said and squatted to show him.

"Good. Now can you squat and extend your left leg?"

I squatted again and extended my left leg.

"Perfect. Yes, you can jump."

I clapped, barely able to contain myself. Since we were beginners, we would jump in tandem—that is, attached to our instructors. We signed up for the photographer package, and they told us where to meet our instructors and when.

Back at the restaurant, Rod was shocked they were allowing me to jump, but there was nothing he could do about it! We spent the remainder of the day watching others jump, land, and repack their parachutes.

We returned to the office and met the photographer. He told us that as soon as we left the plane, we should look straight at him. Sue met the guy she would be jumping with, and he instructed us on what to expect. John, my instructor, didn't arrive until the last minute.

We walked over to the waiting plane, where others were already climbing in. The cabin was no frills, just two long rows of metal benches with seatbelts. It didn't take long before the plane was full. Because of the heat, the main door open was left open. We taxied over to the runway, the engine roaring in our ears. Conversation was impossible. Two solo jumpers sat to my right, next to the open door. Then John and Sue, with her instructor, sat to my left. Across from us was our photographer. As soon as the plane took flight, I leaned over to Sue and yelled, "No turning back now! The only way down is by parachute." Then we gave each other a thumbs up.

It took us about fifteen minutes to get to the proper elevation. While we ascended, I thought, *What the hell are we doing?* But it was too late to change our minds. The jump leader stood up, signaling it was time. One by one, the solo jumpers left the plane.

John had given me goggles, and I had pulled my hair up into a tight ponytail so that it wouldn't blow in my face during our descent. "We're up," he said. "Release your seatbelt and scoot toward the door." I did that. "Now get directly in front of the door and squat with your left leg extended." I did that as well. He was directly behind me, attached by straps and D-clips. He leaned in and said one last thing. "In a few seconds, I'm going to push you out the door."

That few seconds seemed to last forever. *Push me out of the damn plane already.* And then he did.

The photographer was already outside hovering, ready to take our picture. I looked directly at him as instructed. And then we were free falling, John on top, me attached to him below, both of us facing the ground, holding out our arms like we were flying. And we were. The wind pushed my lips and cheeks back into my face, and the noise cushioned me from the world. I even forgot about John. It was just me and the wind and the sky—and I was flying free. No wonder flying has always been the symbol of freedom, of our highest human aspirations, of our reaching for God. At the same time, I was out of my body and perfectly in tune with it. My scars didn't matter, my broken and battered body felt whole. I felt—glorious.

The free fall went on longer than I thought it would, and my mind turned to the patchwork quilt of the land below. We all have to come to earth eventually.

Then suddenly the parachute snapped open, pulling us into a sitting position. Now I was fully aware of John, since I was virtually sitting on his lap. The wind abated and it went quiet compared to the noise storm of the free fall. Now we drifted gently towards the ground. John told me to grab hold of the brake loops attached to the lines on either side, so I could assist with the landing. When I pulled one of the loops, we spun around. He told me to stop that and pull on the other side as he regained sight into our landing path.

As the landing field rose toward us, as it seemed to me, John said, "Start to run."

I pedaled in the air, then caught the ground with a gentle thump. We had a safe and smooth landing. My beautiful, scarred legs held up just fine. We had to gather our chute and move off the field quickly because Sue and her instructor were right behind us. Their landing was equally smooth.

We both had the biggest smiles as we made our way to Rod and the others, who had been watching from the edge of the field.

"Can you believe that?" I said to Sue. "That was life changing."

"If that wasn't the last flight, I'd jump again," Sue said.

"I'd be right there with you."

"Let's not push it ladies," Rod said, beaming with relief that I was safe and intact.

We laughed. "That was the coolest thing I've ever done," I said.

And we had the pictures and t-shirts to prove it.

We were already planning our next adventures—flying a glider and taking a helicopter ride. I thought it might be interesting to see how my dad felt when he almost fell out of the chopper in Vietnam.

AFTERWORD

Why did I risk jumping from a plane after all I've been through? For a simple reason—I no longer fear death, and because I don't fear death, I don't fear life. I want to live as fully as possible.

This feeling began when the Angel revealed herself to me on the way to Yale New Haven Hospital on the day of the accident, and it has grown steadily since then as I faced each trial put before me. I don't live recklessly, but I have no fear! "For God hath not given us the spirit of fear; but of power, and of love, and of a sound mind" (2 Timothy 1:7).

I believe that all the difficulties in my life have shaped me into the person I am today. I have not only accepted my life, I have embraced the challenges. I'm alive! I choose to be happy and productive. I hold no bitterness and have forgiven all of those who have hurt me in one way or another. I have forgiven myself. If I had skipped any of these challenges, I would not have been ready for the next.

While I was hospitalized after the accident, I started a journal, recording what I was dealing with daily. The journal was quite detailed, and I could write only when I wasn't in a great deal of pain. When I finally came home from the hospital, I used our main computer to keep the journal going. I wrote about some of the most personal, heartfelt, and frustrating things I was dealing with. I wanted to keep my writings private, so I named the file "Magazine Subscriptions." Who's going to open that file?

But now it's time to bring the details into the world, to tell my story. Every person has a story, and to some degree we are our stories. Don't hide. Have the courage to tell your story.

I considered writing this book for many years, but I wasn't sure I wanted my children to know ALL the details of my life. I thought about it, and it came to me that to truly prepare our children to live in this world with all its joys and sorrows, we need to tell them the whole truth. It's not that we lie to our children, exactly, but we leave out too much of the bad stuff. We are all guilty of this. We encourage them to be good, to play with others in harmony, to develop interests and discover talents, and to try their hardest. In return, life will be good to them. But sometimes life isn't fair, and they also need to be prepared for that. We live in an imperfect world. Good health should not be taken for granted. I'm proof of that. Sometimes things don't get better tomorrow.

Faith can get us through it, not because faith is the great equalizer or anything like that, but because choosing faith is choosing to be at peace. When we choose to be a Christian, the Lord is constantly grooming us for bigger things. Sometimes being content in our circumstances is the biggest blessing we can receive. I could never have imagined that a series of unprovoked sexual attacks on the thirteen-year-old me would one day lead me on a journey to my highest self. Nor when I was flat on my back in May of 2002 could I have imagined all the blessings I would receive after the accident.

In the end, I moved forward. Writing my story took twenty years, and in the telling, I relived many painful events on my journey, sometimes with great difficulty, but I kept pushing forward. The more I wrote, the more I remembered. I dictated some of the earliest parts of the book, which my friend Shelley transcribed. Some of the details were so painful to remember that I sweated profusely in an air-conditioned house, got sick, and couldn't tape anything for weeks afterwards. This happened while I was writing too. For one two-week period I was writing about such difficult things I had an endless stream of nightmares and ripped off my eyelash extensions while I slept. I had to wear winter gloves to bed to stop doing that. It was good that I continued to see my therapist throughout all this.

In reliving this pain and fear, I was able to overcome it. I learned that I didn't have to be afraid any longer. My brain had been hijacked by fear for too many years. I didn't realize that I held the key to escape. Writing this book has allowed me to release that fear, to bear witness to what happened to me in order to heal, to be honest and authentic. Each word I typed moved me closer to healing, to feeling whole again. Writing this book has been very cathartic. It helped me to let go and let God.

I know that there are far too many women who have experienced sexual abuse and, like me for a long time, haven't been able to tell anyone. I hope that my story will empower you to begin that journey. I cannot begin to tell you how good you will feel when you conquer your fears and demons head on.

Being positive is a choice, not a gift.

The fact that I chose to be a nurse and lovingly care for others was never a surprise to me. The fact that I always dreamed of being a mom, even as a small child, was never a surprise to me. The fact that I ended my career caring for elementary school children was not a surprise to me either, but I am sad that it had to end so quickly. The fact that the Lord has used me in extraordinary ways to help others never surprised me. I know He will continue to use me this way.

We each have our own unique perspective; we were never intended to feel or interpret things the same as anyone else, and that's okay. That's good, even. It would be boring for us to all be the same. Don't compare yourself to others. Learn to appreciate others for their differences. We all have the capacity to grow and learn from the experiences of others, as well as our own. But that, too, is a choice!

Listen more, talk less. Laugh. A lot. Be honest. Only make promises you can keep. Show love and compassion to everyone you meet. Good friends are rare, so treat them like gold. Don't judge others. That's the Lord's job. Listen to good music and sing along. Listen for the tender voice of Jesus whispering in your ear. Simplify, simplify, simplify. Forgive others throughout your earthly stay. By doing so, you will achieve the highest and best form of yourself.

Live your life as I try to do now, without fear! Life is far too short not to enjoy each moment. Enjoy life's ride! God bless you.

NOTES

1. "History of Fort Riley and 1st Infantry Division, accessed October 3, 2022, https://home.army.mil/riley/index.php/about/history."

2. Hazelden Betty Ford Foundation, "Stages of Alcoholism," March 13, 2019, accessed October 9, 2022, https://www.hazeldenbettyford. org/articles/stages-of-alcoholism.

3. D.W. Winnicott, *The Maturational Processes and the Facilitating Environment: Studies in the Theory of Emotional Development* (London: Taylor and Francis, 1995).

4. Shelley J. Kitchura Nelson, "Confidences," Syracuse, NY, unpublished poem, 2013.

5. Joan Anderson, *A Year by the Sea: Thoughts of an Unfinished Woman* (New York: Crown, First Broadway Books Edition, 2000).

6. Eleanor Roosevelt, *You Learn by Living: Eleven Keys for a More Fulfilling Life* (New York: Harper Perennial, Reprint edition, 2016).

7. Elizabeth Kubler-Ross, MD, *Death: The Final Stages of Growth* (New York: Scribner, 1997).

8. International Classification of Diseases (11th ed.), World Health Organization, April 2019. Retrieved November 5, 2019.

9. Peter A. Levine and Ann Frederick, *Waking the Tiger: Healing Trauma* (Berkeley: North Atlantic Books, 1997).

10. Michael John Poirier, "Healing after the Choice," 1994, lyrics used with permission, accessed October 3, 2022, https://www.leavealighton.org.

ACKNOWLEDGMENTS

I never realized that to write a book required a complete team of experts! Without your help, love and support, it would not have been possible for me to accomplish this most important endeavor. So, I am grateful to all of you.

My girlfriend Shelley J. Kitchura Nelson became my first editor. She worked for over four years, first transcribing my dictation, and eventually, editing my work. I never told her about her role in the book, nor how she empowered me and made me realize that I no longer feared my rapist! This reality was tough for her to process. Thanks, Shelley, for your friendship, love, support, dedication, and all your help to bring this important project to fruition.

A special acknowledgement to Raymond Duke Sipherd, a three-time Emmy Award-winning writer. He heard my life story and desperately wanted to become my ghost writer, as well as my second editor. He had great aspirations for this project; however, he passed before any of this was possible. I'm sorry that The Lord had other plans for you, Raymond. Thank you for what you were able to convey to me. I hold onto those dreams as well! Rest in Peace, my friend.

Thanks to my publisher, Laura Bush, for all your expertise, assistance, coaching, and encouragement, especially during my lengthy writer's block last winter. I've gotten to know you quite well since our introduction in 2010 and consider you among my list of friends. Your workshops were always informative and fun to attend. Pilates is also always better when you are there!

A special thank you to Charles Grosel, who completed two edits on my book, including a deep edit. You made my story so much more interesting and readable without losing my voice in the process! Thank you, Charles.

Thanks to Jena Gribble for listening to my vision for the book cover and for your artistic talents in designing it. You've even incorporated symbolism into the designs! Your guidance and expertise have been invaluable!

I also want to thank my girlfriends because you ALL listened with the ears that only true friends possess. Despite my pain, frustration, and crying for answers, you listened without judgment, and you always gave me sound advice, encouraged me, and prayed for me. All of that helped me again and again. I will never forget what any of you did or said to help me. Many of you drove me to appointments and surgeries, which involved hours of your time, but you never complained. Saying "thank you" isn't enough, but I promise that I will never turn my back on any of you either.

A special thanks to Sue for her spontaneity and her willingness to accompany me on my challenges. When sky diving wasn't enough, we tried soaring in a glider. Our next adventure will be flying in a helicopter. With me and Sue, the sky's the limit, so we'll probably always seek thrilling adventures.

Thank you also to my large extended family for your unending support and prayers. I will always miss those of you that have passed, like my mom and dad, my father-in-law, and my mother-in-law. You never were able to witness me completely healed, but you all shaped me into the person that I am today! Thanks for all that you've done.

Thank you to the doctors, nurses, aides, and therapists that took care of me and saved my life and limbs during some of my darkest of days. Also, thanks to all the doctors that cared for me after my mastectomy. They always encouraged me to start my business. Your expertise, advice, patience, skills, compassion, and dedication are the gifts that helped me and others along the way to heal. I will never forget any of you!

Thanks to all the communities that we've been a part of over the years. Your support, unending prayers, food, meals, gift certificates, time, and talent meant so much to me and my family. You came through for us again and again. We will never forget your acts of kindness. We witnessed God in each one of you as you helped us in our times of need.

Lastly, thank you Garrett Moore, for listening to me. You always offered sound advice and guided me through some of my darkest times. I know that you empathetically and sympathetically read every letter that I addressed to you over the years. It always warms my heart to hear your voice on the phone. You will always be the voice for others since you are the best of the best in your field! Thank you, Garrett!

ABOUT THE AUTHOR

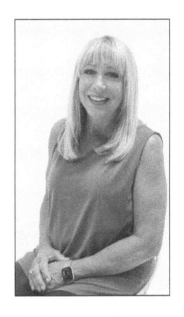

Originally from Pennsylvania, Kim spent her youth traveling across the country with her father's military career. She earned an associate's degree in nursing and business administration, then launched her own career as a critical care RN for over fifteen years. When her husband Rod got the opportunity to run a metals company, the family moved to Connecticut, where Kim became an elementary school nurse.

In 2002, a freak accident ended Kim's very public nursing career. Her book reveals the numerous traumas she has overcome, including confinement to a wheelchair for five years (she had been a runner), fifty-one surgeries to save her life and limbs, and another fifty surgeries after a bilateral mastectomy to treat breast cancer in 2009.

Kim has used her talents and faith to move beyond every obstacle, even starting Miss Daisy Medical, a successful business Kim founded with her doctors' encouragement and input, so she could sell her innovative medical bandages to thousands of patients in need.

Kim would love to hear from you!
Please contact her at kimshipe.com

Checkout Kim's colorful, bacteria-resistant
medical bandages at missdaisymedical.com

CPSIA information can be obtained
at www.ICGtesting.com
Printed in the USA
JSHW020738210623
43508JS00001B/2